IV KETAMINE
INFUSION THERAPY
FOR
DEPRESSION

Why I Tried It, What It's
Like, and If It Worked

Frank M. Ligons, MS

Foreword by Henry H. Macler, MD

The information contained in this book is based upon the research and personal and professional experiences of the authors. It is not intended as a substitute for consulting with your physician or other healthcare provider. Any attempt to diagnose and treat an illness should only be done under the direction of a healthcare professional.

The publisher and authors do not advocate the use of any particular healthcare protocol but believe the information in this book should be available to the public. The publisher and authors are not responsible for any adverse effects or consequences resulting from the use of the ideas or procedures discussed in this book. Should the reader have any questions, they must consult a professional healthcare advisor.

ISBN: 978-1-7368925-1-0 (paperback)

IV Ketamine Infusion Therapy for Depression: Why I Tried It, What It's Like, and If It Worked.

Next Gen Medical, LLC
139 East Main Street
#735
Carnegie, PA 15106

Developmental editor: Amber Hatch
Copy editor: Sarah Lamb
Proofreading: Kaitlin Travis and Kathryn Besaw

This book may be purchased for education, business, or sales and promotional use. For information, please email Find Ketamine at Info@FindKetamine.com.

DEDICATION

Three of the most difficult aspects of severe, chronic illness are the long waits, tough decisions, and financial struggles. Transcending these struggles requires the support and wisdom of family, friends, and medical personnel.

I dedicate this book to all of the insightful, patient, and generous people who made sure that I haven't had to face those challenges alone.

Most specifically, I dedicate this to my dear friend, mentor, and second father, Joseph J. Kennedy III, who spent countless hours saving me from my illness and myself. Joe, I miss your inimitable style, extraordinary intellect, and outrageous humor. You deserve to be here for this.

Dear Reader,

I'm Frank, a 25-year survivor of Treatment-Resistant Depression.

This book tells the story of how Ketamine helped me climb out of crippling depression to **break free from suicidal thoughts**.

But, even without those thoughts, my own habitual ways of thinking and believing held me back from more joy and stability.

I had to learn **different ways of thinking to keep from sliding back into the pit**.

Now, I want to "pay it forward" and help you reach your full potential and stay there.

I'm developing a program that helps **STOP the frustrating backslides into depression** by instilling new ways of thinking that keep your recovery on track.

If you are determined to put depression behind you and move forward with a **permanently** healthier mindset, please reach out to me: Coach@FindKetamine.com.

I try to respond to every inquiry, but few slots are ever open for this 1-on-1 coaching.

Please enjoy this book. My sincere hope is that you and your loved ones find new hope within its pages.

Most Sincerely,

Frank M. Ligons
The Ketamine Coach

TABLE OF CONTENTS

FOREWORD

Henry H. Macler, MD is a board-certified anesthesiologist with over 40 years of experience with Ketamine, first as an anesthetic and later as the adjunct treatment discussed in this book.

Dr. Macler graduated *cum laude* from Albany Medical College and completed his residency in anesthesiology at Peter Bent Brigham Hospital, Harvard University.

Since that time, Dr. Macler has spent decades as the Chief of Anesthesia Services, Chief Quality Officer, and Director of ICU, among other roles at hospitals nationwide.

In these positions, he earned numerous honors, appointments, and awards, including Chief Resident at Peter Bent Brigham Hospital, Harvard University Medical Center, Outstanding Alumni Award from Albany Medical College, and St. Louis University's "The Humanitarian Award," for 18 years of medical service to Haiti and Ukraine.

Pittsburgh Ketamine, founded and directed by Dr. Macler, emerged from a partnership with Dr. Glen Brooks, a pioneer in IV Ketamine infusion therapies at New York Ketamine.

Between the two of them, they have administered over 10,000 Ketamine treatments.

December 2020

Millions of people suffer from depression. Unfortunately, many are "treatment-resistant" and unable to find relief. The outcomes of these cases can be catastrophic.

After witnessing the ravages of mental illness within my own family, I began looking outside of the conventional treatments. That is when a colleague and friend, Dr. Glen Brooks, told me about low-dose IV Ketamine. His successes with Ketamine therapy in New York impressed me deeply. So much so that I opened a branch in Pittsburgh.

Not only did this revolutionary therapy help my family but also over 500 patients through the more than 4,000 treatments conducted at my clinic.

My privilege is sharing in the "understanding moments" of my patients when Ketamine unlocks long-closed doors of insight and satisfaction. From my experience, Ketamine treatments can greatly enhance quality of life and create new momentum in a patient's other therapies. Each day, my "front-row seat" to these transformations encourages and enheartens me.

Rarely do physicians have the opportunity to participate in revolutionary treatments. I count myself incredibly fortunate to play a role in these innovations.

Frank M. Ligons, this book's author, came to me for help two years ago after decades of intense suffering. He and I developed a partnership that, as Frank reports below, changed his life. Our doctor-patient collaboration that led to his success exemplifies what makes my professional life so rewarding.

I hope this book opens a window into the unique therapeutic journey that he and I took together. I believe that both patients and clinicians will benefit from reading this story.

I recommend this publication to my patients, particularly those orienting themselves to this breakthrough treatment and its many possibilities.

Henry H. Macler, MD

INTRODUCTION

Dear Reader,

I've spent most of my life bouncing between working hard and failing harder. Depression, bipolar disorder (BPD), and obsessive-compulsive disorder (OCD) have been brutally consistent companions for decades. Like many of us, my life has been a long trail of diagnoses, disability, and destruction.

To fight these health battles, I've become an expert in advocating for myself through research. For thousands of hours, I've poured over therapies from around the world in every niche I could find.

There aren't many therapies I haven't tried, conventional and alternative alike. My lifetime medical bills have topped $1.4 million (that's $1,400,000). That includes paying for multiple legitimate practitioners, with a few expensive quacks mixed in, but does not factor in the years of lost wages due to my disabled status.

This cycle left me with ballooned weight, dashed hopes, and withered confidence in my future.

Then, I heard about low-dose intravenous Ketamine infusions.

After more than a year of research, I came to believe that this revolutionary therapy, while unlikely to hurt me, had a good chance of helping me.

In my case, *Ketamine came through on both accounts.*

These newfound Ketamine treatments freed me from my daily thoughts of suicide.

They changed my life.

Treatment-resistant depression (TRD) is that which fails to respond to first-line medications. Sufferers of TRD, like myself, are stranded in the darkness of long-term depressive episodes and even suicidal thoughts.

The good news is that low-dose IV Ketamine therapy lifts depression in ***two-thirds*** of these cases.

This book walks you through each step in my decision-making process, from skepticism and desperation to experiencing an innovative treatment and reporting my results.

Why listen to me? I have:

- 25 years of fighting mental health challenges.
- endured numerous stints on disability.
- completed over 20 IV Ketamine treatments, documented with video and personal notes.
- a graduate education with a Master's of Science in Biomedical Informatics.
- analyzed the clinical studies and medical literature.

Join me as I share with you what I've learned about a life-saving treatment, perhaps the biggest breakthrough in the treatment of depression in over 50 years!

Readers will enjoy:

- an easy-to-understand, step-by-step guide to exploring Ketamine as a therapy for severe depression.
- insight into a Ketamine patient's perspective from research to results.
- relief from endless Googling.
- information to speed up the evaluation of this new, life-saving treatment.
- guidance on how to save time and confusion while considering Ketamine.

Who can afford to waste another day in unnecessary agony? Take action! Don't wait!

Life is too short and too precious to spend another day suffering needlessly.

Never give up hope for better tomorrows!

Frank M. Ligons, MS

WHO IS THIS BOOK FOR?

A re you considering Ketamine?
Is it for you?

I don't know. But I do know that more people need to hear about what it can do for them.

Optimism about Ketamine's surprising medicinal benefits is on the rise since its possibilities inspire newfound hope for hard-to-treat conditions.

If nothing you've tried for depression has made a lasting difference, you may have treatment-resistant depression. Ketamine's track record with treating this condition is astonishing, as *two-thirds* of patients report success.

This book is a step-by-step guide to initial research, talking to one's doctor, finding a Ketamine clinic, enjoying the low-dose IV Ketamine therapy treatment experience, and exploring your new life.

This book answers your questions about Ketamine:

- What is it?

- Is it safe?
- What is it like?
- Does it work?
- Where do I find it?

WHO NEEDS THIS BOOK?

- Anyone interested in Ketamine, a breakthrough antidepressant treatment
- People who've tried everything for depression without success and feel like giving up
- Sufferers ready to consider innovative treatments
- Caretakers, parents, and friends considering Ketamine for a loved one
- Providers seeking insight into the Ketamine patient's process of decision-making, concerns, and needs

WHAT WILL YOU LEARN?

- How 25 years of mental health challenges drove me to Ketamine
- How this astonishing treatment provides new hope for depression and other conditions
- Answers to your questions about Ketamine's safety and side effects
- Why a medically educated patient decided to try low-dose IV Ketamine therapy and report his results

- How to talk to your doctor about Ketamine treatments
- What to expect during your Ketamine clinic visit
- If the low-dose IV Ketamine therapy experience is fun or frightening
- About K-holes and bad "trips" - what they are and how to avoid them
- How to be safe and enjoy your therapy
- Tips for a great experience
- What it is like to "feel better"

This guide is written from the patient's perspective to make considering Ketamine easier.

It explains what low-dose IV Ketamine therapy is and why it's drawing attention as a powerful antidepressant.

It documents every step I used in my decision-making process.

You'll hear about the terrible depression symptoms that drove me to find Ketamine.

I'll share the surprising facts I learned about Ketamine's efficacy and safety.

You will discover how to find a good Ketamine clinic and have a useful consultation.

Next, I'll take you step-by-step through the infusion procedure itself, covering the steps of the process and the psychological experience.

You'll get first-hand insight into Ketamine "trips" and the dreaded "K-hole" experience.

You'll get all of my tips to ensure a good treatment experience. These are the tips I wish I had!

Ketamine's benefits in my life are amazing. As someone who has lived and continues to live through this life-changing process, I'll also talk about expectations and what it means to "feel better."

KETAMINE BROUGHT ME BACK FROM THE DEAD

What is it like to "feel dead?"

I don't mean near-death experiences.

I mean, when you feel dead inside. Dead to joy. Dead to hope.

This kind of death is not a happy dream of angels. It's hell.

It's dark, frightening, and everlasting.

If you're reading this, you may know this feeling all too well. And if you know, you sympathize with those enduring the harsh realities of serious illness.

Every one of us carries burdens. Some burdens are visible. Others are not.

I don't mind telling you: I've been through many periods that I found almost impossibly difficult. These times stretched on and on and on. I can't believe I've survived this long.

Ketamine has restored my hope for a better future, not only for myself but for others suffering from severe depression.

I still take life in bite-sized pieces, day by day. But I'm now much more confident that I'll make it. And after all these decades of suffering, this feels like a miracle!

My wish is for all of us to find new hope. Let us all look forward to better tomorrows.

But first, let me tell you about my depressing yesterdays.

IT'S NOT FAIR

My maternal grandmother took her own life when I was only two. With it, we lost her extraordinary kindness, the reassurance of her embrace, and the opportunity to create more memories.

When a life is lost to suicide, you try to make sense of it.

How did this happen?
Why?
Could it have been avoided?
Most painfully, what did I miss?

After all, she had a psychiatrist, a loving trio of daughters, a stable husband, and a talent for baking desserts.

Her psychiatrist rejected her family's concerns. And her husband failed to recognize her decline.

My mom's older sisters had already married and left home, leaving my mother and grandmother to interact as best friends, even sharing clothes and jewelry.

Those exchanges were about to end.

The only warning of my grandmother's passing was one cryptic statement she made to my mother. The day before she left us, instead of planning the usual return of her jewelry, she instead said: "Honey, please take this bracelet. I won't need it anymore."

When my mother found her with the car running, filling the small garage with carbon monoxide, devastation rippled through the family.

A life lost to suicide feels incredibly unjust. It seems so senseless and unnecessary. It's even more jarring when it happens with a well-loved person that "seemed fine."

Could this tragedy have been prevented?

I don't know. But low-dose IV Ketamine therapy helps patients climb out from depression's darkest pits.

She may have been one of them.

TOO MANY DIAGNOSES

Like many other people, my life began with physical health problems: asthma, allergies, strep throat, and bronchitis -- all of which disappeared upon adulthood.

Then came the mental health trouble as I began suffering from obsessive-compulsive disorder (OCD), generalized anxiety disorder (GAD), and social anxiety disorder (SAD).

Beginning in medical school, I was diagnosed with bipolar disorder (BPD) Type 2.

Next, I barely survived a mysterious encephalitis condition (Hashimoto's Encephalitis).

I've no doubt forgotten some diagnoses along the way. It's a long list!

Symptoms from all of these conditions compromise normal function and can lead to awkward and regrettable life effects. Sufferers of medical conditions often endure humiliations related to their illness.

HOW EMBARRASSING

We all need social support, even more so when we're battling a serious illness. That's why it's so cruel when disease cuts into the social bonds we need to recover.

Grinding social anxiety made me avoid people. I can't count the times I've bowed out of a business lunch, rescheduled dinners, or called off from that job.

People noticed.

Some colleagues understandably developed a negative opinion of me. To them, I was disrespectful for blowing them off. I'm sure that's how I came across. My impulse to isolate myself left others feeling rejected.

How could they understand I was hiding from my own problems?

Like many chronically ill people, I tended to self-isolate. I became "Mr. No Show," breaking appointments and avoiding everyone because I felt sick all the time. This tendency led to me falling out of touch with people, ducking out on friends and family, and crawling into a cocoon. Anything to escape more pain, stress, and embarrassment.

Many of us are involuntary "no shows."

Some of us lock ourselves in the house for a year at a time.
Some of us are in the hospital a lot.
Others are on medications that make us emotionally flat and sedate.

All of these circumstances can prevent one from "showing up."

BOOM AND BUST

I've noticed a "boom and bust" pattern in my life.
Work hard.
Bust.
Get good grades.
Bust.
Take a semester off. Wander. Consult with new doctors. Begin moving forward.
Bust.
Medicate myself into semi-functional mush.

Graduate.
Get a good job.
Bust.

Loss of dignity.
Loss of confidence.
Disability status.

I just keep repeating this cycle.
Does any of this sound familiar to you?

Let me share with you one of the most impactful moments of my life when my diagnoses turned a harmless experience into a personal horror.

CORNERED

My father spent numerous post-retirement years singing in nursing homes, bringing joy to thousands of residents who magically came back to life as they sang songs from their early days. During one of my periods of disability, my dad suggested I try to get back on my feet by coming out to his jobs with him. He'd have me do little things like setting up his equipment: speakers, cables, microphones. Occasionally, he'd even push me into singing a bit myself.

The first day I accompanied him on his job, I recall my panic clearly. We had just moved his sound equipment into the meeting room. Nursing aides wheeled in the audience. Residents came in all conditions, some able-bodied but unable to live independently. Some were physically disabled and contorted by arthritis, strokes, and neurological disorders. Bearing witness to all of the different medical circumstances in that room utterly overwhelmed me.

As an OCD sufferer with health-based ruminations, this room contained all of my worst nightmares.

My dad asked me to help set up the equipment, run some speaker wire, and test the microphone. Of course, I'd have to go into "the room" to do it. I'd have to brush past wheelchairs, avoid soiled clothing, and stay ever vigilant about how precisely I moved to avoid "contamination." To my horror, in this already panicked state, one of the residents grabbed me and tried to kiss me on the mouth!

That day, as the show was about to start, I wanted to be in the room helping. But fear took me hostage. I struggled against incapacitation. I felt panicky. Keep in mind that I was already unable to work. I had just spent a year locked in my house. Here was my first attempt to get back into the real world. My mind filled with visions of catastrophic medical disasters.

I was gasping for air, thoughts ablaze; I prayed for peace as terrifying imaginations of the patients in the next room closed in. Visions of being "in their shoes" made me shudder. How would I endure in that condition? I found it hard to look at the audience. I did, though, and someone caught my eye.

There was a young gentleman in the back of the room. He wasn't anywhere near retirement age. He may have been in his 20s. The staff wheeled him in with a heavy-duty chair. Because he was young, he still had a good bit of weight to him. His chair had a headrest to support his involuntarily twisted neck.

Rather than an open lap that allowed the passenger to stand up, his thighs braced a little desk, like the ones used by school children. Somehow, his condition had him bent towards the desk. That's why it was there: to give his arms something to lean on. From what I could tell, he had little control over his limbs. He looked taut and frozen. I felt tragically horrible for this man. Surely, no one deserved a lifetime of this. Even 20 years later, I can still see him.

Hiding in the hallway, I had a decision to make. Rationally, I knew that going back in wouldn't hurt me. There was nothing contagious there. We would perform, pack up the truck, and return to a less distressing home life.

But anxiety doesn't work that way. It scoffs at rationality. I shook in that hallway with its blue cinder block walls, its well-meaning end tables with fake flowers. They weren't soothing. This place embodied the stark horrors of my worst fears.

My mind would not release the obsession with ending up like that poor young man in the back of the room. I kept thinking about the proximity of the bathroom. How far away was the sink where I could wash my hands? But then, who else washed their hands there? Residents? Staff? Could I wash off my fears in there?

But we all know the answer to that. It's not easy to wash away fears, wash away worry, wash away that depressed feeling. You've likely tried. I know I did. Eventually, it feels like you run out of options, but that is why I'm here to reassure you that there might be another way.

THE WORKIN' BLUES

When I came out of undergrad, I got a great job with an international consulting firm. Newfound freedom from schooltime poverty and late-night cram sessions promised a celebration of new friends and fortune (well, not quite "fortune," but it felt like that). My colleagues and I, us "new recruits," bonded over hard work and new responsibilities. Even with my health problems, this new world's excitement fueled my professional and social ambitions.

We traveled all week for work. We sipped on fancy cocktails we charged to clients or could finally afford on our own. Despite whatever benefits that we enjoyed, we continued the long-time tradition of complaining about our bosses.

Around a year and a half in, my issues of anxiety and depression ground me down. I was a disaster, physically and emotionally, from this high-pressure, high-flying lifestyle. While my friends would occasionally turn tired or frustrated, I was becoming overwhelmed and unstable.

My doctors increased my medications. Eventually, I couldn't wake up in the morning. Instead of being there at 8 am, like my peers, I'd drag myself in at 10 am. Can you imagine the heat I was getting from "upstairs?" Here I was, this young upstart, showing up for work TWO HOURS LATE every day! Was I nuts?

My managers weren't impressed. And, let's face it, I looked perfectly healthy on the outside. They knew I was qualified to do the work. They could only conclude that I was irresponsible and disrespectful, breeding resentment and negative feedback. This unfortunate cycle stimulated even more anxiety and depression. My mind spun like a revolving door of unlikely catastrophes to the point of incapacitation. My mood became frail and fatalistic. Eventually, my whole being collapsed. I felt like my life was over. I called Human Resources and told them I needed time off. I never made it back.

Losing that job wasn't the most troublesome aspect I faced; it was losing my friends. I had some good friends in the firm that meant a lot to me. But my frequent meltdowns were untenable. I heard from friends less and less. All they knew was that I disappeared one day and ended up on long-term disability.

Twenty years isn't that long ago, but mental health challenges were still more stigmatized and misunderstood than they are now. I couldn't do a great job of explaining myself either. Plus,

I was taking a barrage of meds. Who knows what I said or did to the people around me as I fell off the map?

One particular night, I recall talking to a friend and asking for his support as I attempted to change my life for the better. Whether I was speaking gibberish or whether he wanted nothing to do with the drama, I still remember the feeling of an impenetrable wall rising between us.

Think back to your relationships: family, friends, and colleagues. Do any of my experiences sound familiar?

WILL THEY STICK WITH ME?

Many of us have loved ones with health problems. We want to care for them and fulfill their needs, but it's complicated. Sometimes, the overwhelming exhaustion of being a caregiver strains a relationship past the breaking point, which is natural and understandable. It's difficult for both parties. This dynamic reminds me of a particular case when I was in a new and promising relationship.

I was already having health problems before meeting her, and I told her about them. She was very caring and understanding. When I would lock myself in after work each day, she would sit on the couch with me, glued to "The First 48." I felt accepted. I felt like, here's a girl who is OK with me as I am. Our future doesn't depend upon me miraculously transforming into this perfectly healthy person to improve our relationship.

During that time, I agonized every minute of the day. My medications were giving me akathisia, and I was screaming inside. This inhuman pain burned my entire body and brain. There was a spear sticking through my skull. My nervous system was hooked up to a battery, overloading my pain sensors and causing me to tremor. My neck was tight. My jaw clenched. I felt like if I stopped moving, I would jump out the window.

I still went to work. Intense exercise during lunch and after work provided some relief. I'd hit the gym on my lunch break. Then, the raft of meds I was on would put me to sleep. Lunchtimes, post-gym, you'd find me passed out in my car at the far end of the parking lot. My colleagues didn't know what to think. My late arrivals, furtive dashes off to the gym, and naps in the parking lot didn't bring scores of new friends.

After work, I would drive downtown, rip my bike from the trunk, and pedal the trails as fast as possible. When I pedaled hard enough, for long enough, I could feel the electrification of my nervous system withdrawal. While I never became completely calm, I could survive another day.

My new girlfriend was a tremendous supporter. She listened to me, brainstormed medical decisions, and comforted me through the text messages we exchanged throughout the day. At night, we watched goofy reality TV shows, followed by her tucking me in.

Getting into bed, I could sense my body beginning to writhe. Muscles were tightening. Adrenaline began pumping. Trying to lay down and "rest" was laughable under these circumstances. That's why her waiting with me to sleep every night was so helpful. She would climb into bed and listen for me to lapse into sleep. Then, she would gracefully sneak out and head back home. She did this every night. Even now, I look back upon her devotion with awe.

However, there did come a day when she couldn't do it anymore.

After an evening meal at my place, the break unfolded. I was no doubt squirming from my daily bout of burning alive. I slumped into my usual needy state. It was the last straw.

Understandably distraught, she vented her long pent-up frustrations. She confessed to being worn out from taking care of me. It was just too much and too constant and everlasting. Given my fragility and having a definite appreciation for her essential role in my daily life, this was frightening and disheartening.

I understood, though. I conceded her right to be exhausted, burnt to a crisp. How couldn't she be? I felt the same way about taking care of myself! I wish I could've walked away *with* her.

Of course, I felt dejected. I wasn't mad *at her*. I just knew I would miss her. The word "miss" didn't capture it. She was the bridge to my remaining slivers of social function. Once again, my substandard health was destroying my relationships. That was a 1-2 punch.

I've spent years on disability. I've been barricaded alone in my house. I've watched in angry despair as my hard-won earnings disappeared into doctors' pockets. I've watched friends walk away. Girlfriends trail off. Colleagues snicker.

Do you know anyone that can relate to this? It's a difficult downfall.

The "Frank" of years ago would've been too embarrassed to confess these stories. But, as other people have inspired me with their honesty, it's my turn to throw out a lifeline.

I hope you will take these confessions as a way to connect with me. So, when I say there is hope and help (even if it's not Ketamine), you can say, "OK, maybe. Frank sounds like a bad case. If he's optimistic, I can be too."

JUST TRY HARDER

Carrying a medical burden is expensive: financially, emotionally, and socially.

Have you lost friends? Been unfairly judged?

Maybe you've just drifted away because of your isolation?

Lost a job? A spouse? Custody of your children? Or just some self-respect?

When you can't "snap out of it" or "take a pill," *you* are the most frustrated. You feel terrible watching the movie of your life starring you as the sick, lonely, and misunderstood character.

These backslides are not from the lack of trying--just the opposite. I've put my very best into every effort. For many years, not just days or weeks, I've pushed myself beyond the breaking point. But in life, as we all know, you don't always get an "A" for effort. Instead of comparing myself to others, I remind myself that whatever my achievements, I've made them despite my soul-sucking illness.

Even as the public becomes more educated, people often don't "get it." But *I get it.* I know how mentally and physically excruciating a health problem can be.

While depression is somewhat relatable to the general public, with most people having a sense of what it feels like to be "sad," bipolar disorder and OCD are more abstract.

Here's an example from my own life:

Do you know that quick email you dash off to a friend or colleague? That may take me hours. I can't stop checking it, reading it, rereading it, rechecking it, squinting at it, and reconsidering it.

When I'm cleaning, I engineer an ordering of tasks that will be the least "contaminating." I wouldn't want to schedule brushing my teeth after touching that filthy garbage can.

Whenever I hear or see a date, my mind launches into calculations. If that movie came out in 1991, how old was I? If someone was born in the same year but a different month, how far apart are our ages? Am I older or younger than them?

Am I going to lose control of myself or my thoughts and do something rash or illegal? Will I end up in jail without a defense even I can understand?

When are my loved ones and friends going to die? Which one(s) will die first? Can it be prevented? Will I survive their parting?

These are standard daily obsessions in my life. There are many more. They overrun my mind from morning to night. Do they then rest? No. Sleep brings vivid night terrors.

Is it any wonder how a person's mental health suffers? Do you ever experience some of these thoughts? That spiral, that frantic and endless churning of your worries and fears?

It's tough to live in this kind of mental state. To watch everyone else, seemingly fine and happy, going through life "effortlessly" while you can barely get out of bed or take out the trash.

I'm confessing some of my baggage here in hopes you'll feel more comfortable reading along. We all need some encouragement. When someone shows vulnerability, it is a reminder that we are not alone. That someone imperfect, just like the rest of us, is making progress.

Most of my health concerns are psychiatric. Low-dose IV Ketamine therapy's impact on mental and behavioral health conditions is what I know the most about as a researcher and a patient. Accordingly, the text below refers to these conditions often. The good news is that people are finding help for other conditions, including forms of chronic pain and substance abuse.

WHAT DO I DO NEXT?

NOW WHAT?

O nce you feel trapped in a chronic, severe illness, you have three options:

1) Accept your suffering.
2) Die.
3) Continue the excruciating quest for better health.

I suck at the first.
I'm scared of the second.
That leaves me with the third.

TAKING THE THIRD

Take (choose) the third option with me.
Not because it's easy. Or that it guarantees happiness.

Take the third because perseverance always brings progress.
Take the third and simply refuse to give up!

ISN'T IT TOO LATE FOR ME?

I can't even remember how many times I've asked myself this same question: when I was 18, 19, 20, 21, 22... even this morning.

Years back, I had an excellent OCD therapist. What he told me sticks in my mind and even makes me laugh sometimes. When I asked him about all of the time I lost to bad health, he said to consider those the "lost years," "years in the void," etc. He chuckled. He wasn't being dismissive or cruel.

He was essentially saying: Frank, you can spend every day pondering all the things you might have lost. He reminded me that contemplating life's missed opportunities doesn't require you to have OCD. We could all sit down and marinate in thoughts of lost possibilities. Try not to get stuck in that. If you can, laugh about it. Laugh about how insane life is, how it takes things away, and how it rarely provides satisfactory answers.

We all carry memories and fantasies about the things we've missed. We mourn the time we've irretrievably lost or wasted. After all, life is finite, and when you add up your times of suffering in terms of years, it can be a long time. Our human lives, no matter what you believe happens next, are always short.

I used to think my circumstances were unique. That I was in a special kind of hell, a place unreasonable and so much worse than anyone else's. Now, I know that all of us feel this way at one time or another. For some people, it's an illness that robs them of joy. Others, it's poverty. Some people have lost loved ones. Some people never had anyone to love.

You may not have my challenges, but you have plenty of your own.

Humans are obsessed with happiness. When we feel unhappy or not happy enough, we ask things like, if I hadn't been sick,

- how rich and prosperous would I have been?
- how much better would it have been if my mom/dad/spouse/sibling had been there?
- would I have wasted so much time making poor decisions?
- would I be healthier, better looking, or more connected?

So, after I ask myself how much of my life has been marred and mangled by mental illness, I try to remember that every life has its imperfections, letdowns, and disappointments. There will always be "what ifs" and "if onlys."

Am I good at accepting this? No.

Redirecting our hearts and minds away from these despairing thoughts is infinitely more comfortable to talk about than put into practice. But it can be reassuring to know that our happiness and sadness are always there. We can focus in on either of them.

Do you ever catch yourself feeling really good? Maybe you're on a walk, and you've forgotten your troubles on a sunny day. Maybe you feel just a bit better today; there's more spring in your step. Perhaps you received a compliment. Got a bonus at work. Found a medicine that takes the edge off.

If you're reading this, you've probably caught yourself feeling bad. Maybe you feel sad. Your mind is full of the memories of everything you've lost. You don't see a way out. No one has an encouraging word. You feel like giving up.

Both the good and the bad days, the happy and the sad thoughts are real. They are both there. One day may have more of one than the other. But, when we make a habit of deciding to live to see more good days than bad, that choice can come true.

Few of us will reach the end of our lives with zero regrets. Few of us will get to lie there smiling about how everything went well, how all our decisions were perfect, and how life just kept coming up roses.

Can we take all of those good and bad days, all of those triumphs and regrets, all of our helplessness, defiance, stubbornness, and poor fortune to fuel something inside us? Maybe the healthiest thing to do, no matter who we are or what our problem is, is to use all of those uncomfortable truths to ignite an even greater zest for life going forward?

You know the part in a movie when the hero gets beaten up and knocked down? He's beaten senseless, bleeding crawling on the ground to escape. But he's not going to make it. Until…there's a new expression developing on his face. It's transitioning from defeat to disgust. To determination. To anger and rebellion and defiance.

He's going to get up and strike back. He's going to muster whatever the very last of himself is. There's not enough pain or defeat or overwhelming odds to keep him down. He's not done. He draws himself up. He's wobbly, unsteady. Maybe he can't see clearly. His foe is bearing down on him. But there's now something forceful about him. Something brave, confident, and terrifying. Now, he's going to strike back. Strike back against his foe, against life, his sickness, his disability, his discouragement. He's going to give as good as he's gotten.

Why is this scene in so many movies? Because everyone can relate. WE ARE the ones knocked down. We are the ones out for the count. Just like the character in the movie, we must summon our last ounce of strength to overwhelm our opponent.

BUT I'VE TRIED IT ALL!

I understand. One of the reasons I kept looking for alternative treatments is that I hate medicine. I take more medications each day than I care to admit.

I literally take medication by the handful.

They cause weight gain. They injure my liver.
Sometimes, I can't go to sleep. Sometimes, I can't wake up.

There are times I can't feel my emotions.

I get irate and frustrated.

I'm worn down and defeated.

From childhood, I've always been dependent on one medication or another. As a baby, I required drugs for asthma and allergies. Then, I would have recurring bouts of bronchitis and strep throat, leading to excessive antibiotics and steroids. By high school, I had chronic fatigue syndrome. At university, I fell into severe OCD and depressive episodes. On two separate occasions, I had to beg for medical leave. I got behind schedule. My friends kept on track.

I've yet to meet someone who wants to be on medicine. But I know a lot of people, including myself, that *need to be* on it. I'm resentful about being such a loyal pharmaceutical customer.

However, the brutal truth is: I wouldn't have made it this far without medication.

Even when the costs were very high in side effects, stigmatization, and finances, the medications still helped. They are a necessary evil in my life. I'd love to be rid of them someday.

Millions of people feel this way. Millions of people hate drugs, their mediocre results, and their intolerable side effects.

I have personally tried almost every relevant psychiatric medication—SSRIs, SNRIs, antipsychotics, beta-blockers, mood stabilizers...and on and on.

I've tried 28 of them.

Typical Antipsychotics
Haldol

Atypical Antipsychotics
Abilify
Risperdal
Seroquel
Zyprexa

Mood Stabilizers
Depakote
Lithium
Lamictal

Tricyclics
Anafranil

Monoamine uptake inhibitors
Celexa
Lexapro
Luvox
Paxil
Prozac
Zoloft
Desyrel
Effexor
Remeron
Serzone
Wellbutrin

Why stop there?

Klonopin
Xanax
Valium
Ativan
BuSpar
Inderal
Serax
Dextromethorphan

Don't get me wrong. Some of these have helped me. Some are still helping me. Despite my frustration with taking them, I know how bad I get without them.

But they take as much as they give.

I'd be lying if I said that my self-esteem doesn't take a hit when I compare my pre-medication size to now. I don't even know when to buy new clothes or just keep the old ones because my weight could be completely different next month.

I recall feeling attractive prior to this new invisibility, ridicule, and disgust. How do I break out of being repelled by my own self?

Let's talk about another aspect of these medications. One that most people don't like to even think about. During the early days of my pharmaceutical treatment, I had the most frustrating and awkward sexual side effects.

Some of us begin these medications when we're young. Often, we are too young to have any excuse for being sexually dysfunctional, too young to keep explaining to our partners why we can't or don't want to perform, and too young to imagine a life without normal sexual expression.

Who even wants to bring it up? Many people don't even tell their doctor. Patients get stuck choosing psychiatric relief with a boatload of side effects versus remaining dysfunctional while being otherwise "normal."

What's the right balance when either scenario is oppressive? Should I trade some sex for feeling suicidal?

What if I stop eating? Will I still gain weight? It sure would be nice not blowing up like a whale.

No problem. I'll quit the meds and end up confined to my house, a hostage to my panic attacks.

Maybe I'll just get no sleep and feel exhausted all the time? That's really productive, right? Managers love a dependably late employee.

Once again, medication can be helpful. It can be the difference between life or death. There are those of us who will always need them. Thankfully, the mediocre track record of these drugs and their depressing side effects are creating more interest in alternative approaches like Ketamine.

CONSIDERING THE ALTERNATIVES

When facing severe health problems and having tried many remedies without success, it can be challenging to keep an open and positive attitude. When you're in pain, *you don't feel* open or positive.

Why would you? You're overwhelmed with no end in sight.

When you are feeling discouraged, that's when it's MOST necessary to investigate alternatives. Commit to the willingness to find healing where least expected. Avoid those who are closed to new approaches. Stubbornness about finding a new way forward is counterproductive. If you are suffering, please don't resign yourself to continuing on the same track of what's not working. Keep learning. Keep searching.

I don't know if Ketamine is for you. But I believe that something out there IS better for you. Keep turning over stones until you find something useful.

I've seen people recover from all kinds of diseases throughout my life and from a wide variety of treatments. One common thread in these breakthroughs is the realization that whatever got them into the disease would NOT get them out. Because of this change in thinking, some of these former sufferers found new solutions and are living better lives than they thought possible!

A few years ago, I began hearing about the drug, Ketamine. I heard it might help treat a variety of mental, physical, and addiction problems. My ears perked up as I sat there, struggling to manage my own chronic health problems. Once I learned of the striking reports of low-dose IV Ketamine's antidepressant activity, I had to investigate.

I started by committing myself to reconsidering my old, outdated thinking about this "club drug" to uncover the truth. It didn't happen all at once. But over time, what I learned completely changed my opinion. I'm so glad it did!

DON'T BELIEVE EVERYTHING YOU READ

Besides my own skepticism, some people told me they thought Ketamine was "snake oil. Stop believing everything you read on the internet."

The phrase "snake oil" stretches back to the 18th century. It refers to bogus remedies peddled to unknowing customers by unscrupulous doctors, pharmacists, and salespeople. But we all know what it means: the stuff is garbage. It won't help. It may even hurt. They're just selling it to make money.

It's easy to relegate new or little-known health treatments to the category of "snake oil." After all, questionable remedies always circulate around those desperate for help. But can I afford to dismiss everything out of hand? I DO need help. I can't get too negative. I can't afford to start reflexively saying, "Oh, that's bull, that's bogus."

Just because one thing may not work out, we can't just start saying "no" to everything. Life has risks. People usually focus on the risk of doing something. But another risk is NOT doing something. Experimentation can produce unexpected results.

HOW I CHOSE KETAMINE

CONSIDERING KETAMINE TREATMENT

F irst, I made an honest assessment.
Every day is a battle.
My quality of life is zero.
I can't function normally in society.

I feel worthless, embarrassed, and humiliated by my condition. Other people's lives are progressing while mine is frozen. Life is short, and I'm missing out on so many good and important things.

I may be surviving. But, *I'm not living.*

Second, I summarized my research.

The "risk to reward" ratio for low-dose IV Ketamine therapy is attractive.
I've taken many more dangerous medications without positive results.

Third, I came up with a comprehensive plan to cover all of the information sources I could find. My approach was to analyze scientific literature, clinical trials, testimonials, competing sides of the issue, risks and safety issues, and the likelihood of helping me with the depressive symptoms of my Bipolar Disorder. I added that to talking with Ketamine clinics for my final decision.

Finally, I decided that if I didn't try, I would never know.

I will walk you through the details of my process below.

TESTIMONIALS AND ANECDOTES

If the word "rumor" has an analogous term in medicine, it is "anecdote." Anecdotal evidence is information that does not come from rigorous, verifiable, and repeatable studies but rather through rumors, patient stories, and aberrant cases. This term bears a negative connotation in the sciences. Because medicine insists on well-designed studies with robust, repeatable results, "rumors" and observations outside of these conditions carry a low value.

It may sound strange coming from someone indoctrinated in the rational, scientific method, but when I feel overwhelmed with symptoms, I go looking for testimonials. Testimonials are the unsung heroes of medical knowledge. Like any information I receive, I don't blindly accept its validity. However, I have found many gems in these stories. Their claims may not yet be backed by clinical evidence, but when you need help, everything is worth looking into.

A stranger's testimony could be your ticket out of misery.

People managing health conditions frequently belong to online and real-life forums and support groups. A lot of valuable "unofficial data" comes from patients in these communities. Unfortunately, the medical industry generally downplays and denies the legitimacy of information from these sources.

For instance, it took years to acknowledge, define, and proactively treat the akathisia side effect sometimes caused by antidepressant use. It is a terrible side effect, capable of driving users to suicide and perhaps even encourage violent behavior directed at others. It also took several years for any official acknowledgment of the severe and widespread nature of drug withdrawal, aka "Discontinuation Syndrome."

Figuring out all of a drug's benefits and risks takes time. Patterns may take years to appear. But these patterns may begin emerging years earlier if one monitors the "unofficial" communication channels. Medical school instills a reflexive dismissive action to the potential importance of such "weak evidence."

After all, what's the value of one person's story from some corner of the internet? Is that person a doctor? What's their expertise? Are they promoting a product? How do you know if they were sick and are now well? And, if they really were helped, how do you know what really helped them? So many questions.

However, anecdotal evidence has one HUGE advantage: under the right circumstances, it can be unusually objective.

During your non-stop Googling, you run across testimonials from people just like you espousing Ketamine's benefits.

They don't appear to be selling anything. They're just reporting on how some "weird" treatment helped them when nothing else could. You start thinking, "Why can't this stuff help me too?"

Your heart beats faster. Hope creeps in.

Word continues to spread. Discussions about low-dose IV Ketamine therapy by both providers and patients are becoming more public. There are tons of YouTube videos and blogs talking about Ketamine's benefits.

Couldn't there be something to that?

So, you look into it.

WHAT I FOUND OUT

Questions remain about who Ketamine will help, under what circumstances it should be prescribed, its risk/reward ratio, and its precise mechanism of action. However, in this book, I'll be sharing my thoughts from being a low-dose IV Ketamine therapy patient and a biomedical research scientist accustomed to scouring medical literature. (Note: I am not a doctor and am not licensed to provide any medical advice. All of your medical conditions and treatments must be addressed by licensed medical personnel only.)

Currently, Ketamine is being used to treat

- mood disorders such as depression, anxiety, OCD, and bipolar disorder.

- severe pain conditions like neuropathy, migraines, and chronic regional pain syndrome.
- addiction to alcohol and opiates.

Any licensed physician is permitted to prescribe and administer Ketamine. Anyone from a psychiatrist to an anesthesiologist has this privilege. However, it is worth noting that anesthesiologists are often the most familiar with Ketamine because it is an anesthetic and therefore within their purview. My low-dose IV Ketamine therapy treatments are administered by an anesthesiologist.

When Ketamine is prescribed for anything else besides anesthesia, we call this "off-label." Many drugs are given for "off-label" uses. This term simply means that a drug is found to have other applications outside of those officially approved by the FDA. It is perfectly legal to prescribe drugs in this manner and is even common practice.

One example of this practice involves a medication called Trazodone. Trazodone is technically an antidepressant, but it is often prescribed for sleep because its dominant side effect is the quick onset of drowsiness.

Ketamine is an old drug whose use dates back to the 1960s. It is an intriguing medication, not only because of its frequent, amazing impact on patients but because of its benign side effect profile. In other words, its risk to reward ratio is very positive. Yes, there are possible complications of low-dose IV Ketamine therapy, but they are mild and include such things as bruising at the IV site, dizziness, and fatigue.

Serious complications are rare. One doctor I know has administered literally thousands of treatments while encountering only a handful of potentially serious complications (easily addressed by on-site equipment), all without injury or death.

Personally, I find these treatments very pleasant and rarely accompanied by unpleasant side effects. And even if one does experience side effects, they pass very quickly (usually within 30–60 minutes post-treatment).

There is sometimes confusion about Ketamine's safety because people refer to the illegal and hazardous use of Ketamine as a recreational drug. The recreational use of Ketamine carries serious potential risks due to factors such as high dosage, overly frequent and chronic use, and variations in the purity of the substance users are purchasing on the black market. One of the reasons low-dose IV Ketamine therapy is so safe is that the treatment doses are lower than those applied to anesthetic situations and dramatically lower than what recreational users consume.

In terms of low-dose IV Ketamine therapy's use and efficacy regarding mental/mood disorders, its preliminary track record is impressive; more impressive than the response rate of antidepressants, and without the typical 2-12 week delay.

It is generally accepted that about two-thirds of patients with treatment-resistant depression experience significant relief. Importantly, this statistic includes suicidal patients who, through Ketamine, can experience an almost miraculous elevation out of that lethal state of mind. As far as I know, there are no other medical interventions that are so immediately and dramatically effective in life-and-death mental health emergencies.

Think how many lives could have been, and will be, saved by a safe treatment that takes only minutes to rescue a person from their suicidal state. As someone familiar with the effects of suicide in my own family, this possible future is incredibly promising.

Regarding chronic pain conditions, Ketamine also shows promise. The statistics for this category of treatment aren't as well known to me. But one aspect of the relief from severe pain is actually psychologically similar to that of the above mood disorders. Chronic pain conditions frequently accompany and/or induce depression and anxiety. Therefore, one might say that receiving a Ketamine infusion for pain/neuropathy offers a 2-for-1 possibility. One may experience both physical and emotional relief from the treatment.

Though not as well known, Ketamine's application to addiction therapy is another avenue of research. Studies on Ketamine's ability to combat addiction were largely pioneered by a Russian physician named Dr. Evgeny Krupitsky, with experiments beginning 40 years ago.

As for how Ketamine works to produce all of the above, our understanding is still unfolding. The most accepted current theory involves NMDA receptors and glutamate. Very generally speaking, this model posits that Ketamine regulates the activity of the glutamatergic system: perhaps by boosting the underactive areas associated with poor emotional status while down-regulating overactive neuronal networks.

There is also talk of neurogenesis, meaning the growth and repair of neuronal connections within the brain. Perhaps the growth of a denser neural network where it is somehow damaged may result in a wide variety of improvements in both physical and mental/emotional functions. If this hypothesis is correct, Ketamine may offer new therapies for traumatic brain injuries and degenerative neurological conditions such as dementia and Alzheimer's.

Although IV Ketamine is a very promising treatment, it will not help everyone. It does not magically repair one's life or do away with one's problems. Its positive effects may manifest within one's first treatment, after many treatments, or never. It is expensive and not routinely covered by insurance. Even when it works, one often needs booster treatments at some interval (generally every month or two).

But, if you have suffered from an agonizing and debilitating condition as I have, you are likely encouraged just by the *possibility* of finding a treatment that works for you.

IS KETAMINE DANGEROUS?

NO EASY ANSWERS

I t took me over a year of research using medical journals, websites, YouTube testimonials, and expert lectures before I felt comfortable on the issue of safety. Ultimately, I couldn't find a dangerous reason to decline giving low-dose IV Ketamine therapy a try. But that decision took me longer than necessary. I didn't have this book pulling all of the information together.

QUESTIONS OF SAFETY

Assessing a drug's safety requires two questions.

1) What is its safety record as reported in clinical trials and from front-line clinics?

As for low-dose IV Ketamine therapy's safety record, based on my research combined with feedback from doctors with more than 10,000 infusions, it is impressive. When I say "impressive," I don't mean that we know all of the long-term effects of Ketamine treatment. It's too early to know. Treatments may even add up to MORE positive results over time. This has been my experience. Continual rebuilding of neural networks is a property of Ketamine motivating research into combating dementia.

Properly administered, critical reactions are rare. With thousands of treatments under his belt, my doctor has encountered only a handful of "emergencies" requiring intervention. Plus, these "emergencies" were benign airway obstructions from apnea.

Side Effects

- Injection site pain
- Dizziness
- Blurred/double vision and nystagmus
- Nausea/vomiting and loss of appetite
- Dreamlike feeling/confusion/unusual thoughts/ hallucinations
- Inflammation of urinary tract/cystitis
- Respiratory disturbances
- Heart arrhythmia, hypotension, and bradycardia
- Seizures/abnormal movements

Ketamine's side effect profile is well-known due to its widespread use over the past 60 years. Its side effects are generally mild, transitory, and dose-dependent.

There is monitoring during a Ketamine infusion, including EKG, pulse, and oxygen levels. The staff will also check on you regularly to ensure you are not experiencing discomfort.

Personally, the only side effects I've ever experienced are tiredness, disorientation, thirst, double vision, and the occasional "unpleasant trip." All of these resolve within an hour or so. Those effects don't stop me. I always feel relaxed after a treatment. Any side effects will be gone soon and won't harm me.

In fact, because the Ketamine experience itself is usually so positive for me, I don't even look at these as "side effects" in a negative way. Basically, when I go for treatment, I know I'm being medicated. I still feel good. And I don't mind whatever short-lived hiccups I may experience.

2) What are the risks of NOT taking treatment?

The costs of depression, whether referring to finances, work functionality, or emotional suffering and instability, are high across every dimension. Therefore, our definition of "safety" must include not only health but the safety of all areas of our lives. Given that, determining whether avoiding a medication is the "safer" choice is not easy. In my mind, when a drug is required to save a life, it is safer than the alternative.

Ketamine with Other Medications

Being someone on numerous medications, I worried that I'd be disqualified from treatment. I discovered that many people receiving Ketamine infusions are also on other medications, including those for psychiatric use. In my personal case, there are a couple of psychiatric medications that my doctor instructed me not to take within a certain number of hours before treatment.

It is critical to inform your doctor of any and all medications, street drugs, and s--upplements you may be taking to ensure safe and effective treatment.

Party On

Ketamine, like any substance, can be both addictive and dangerous. Abusing it may lead to psychological or physical dependency. However, these properties apply almost exclusively to the "recreational user." Ketamine, when used recreationally and in large doses, can cause everything from bladder damage to death; just one reason why it requires a prescription.

When I was researching Ketamine for the first time, I came across crazy stories that were both positive and negative. What I didn't realize at the time was that only a fraction of the negative stories were under normal conditions. Often, when you see a list of serious side effects for Ketamine, it's due to a high dosage either for anesthetic or much more dangerous, recreational purposes.

How are low-dose IV Ketamine treatments different?

- Require a legal prescription
- Minimal doses
- Supervised by medical personnel

Potential for Addiction

Antibiotics are overprescribed. NSAIDs are overused. Opioids are causing a health crisis on an unfathomable scale. Still, when prescribed and used responsibly, all of these medications have their place in the medical toolbox.

Low-dose IV Ketamine therapy should be prescribed and administered with caution. Additional screening is applied to patients with a history of substance abuse. Once dependent, Ketamine addicts may suffer serious withdrawal symptoms, including psychosis.

The risk of addiction increases with recreational use in unsanctioned settings. If you are not in an appropriate medical setting with your vital signs being monitored and under the supervision of a physician qualified to react to any potential adverse effects, you are endangering yourself. Not being in the proper medical setting, even with people you trust, is never "safe." While serious adverse events during Ketamine administration are rare, dangerous reactions could even lead to death without the necessary medical personnel and equipment in place.

WHAT DO I HAVE TO LOSE?

For many people considering low-dose IV Ketamine treatment, there is a desperation for relief that supersedes the anxiety of the unknown, which was true for me. "What did I have to lose?"

was my personal decision after living so many years in crippling pain.

With a predominantly benign side effect profile, I decided I was trading little risk for a shot at a large reward. After all, in my mind, the long-term use of medications and their side effects represent a much more serious threat to my health, particularly in the long term.

Time to talk things over with my doctor.

CONSULTING A DOCTOR ABOUT KETAMINE

TALKING WITH YOUR PHYSICIAN

D octors in numerous fields are enthusiastic about Ketamine's prospects. Its breakthrough potential regularly garners media attention.

Leading up to your consultation, prepare your questions in advance. Then, you will be relaxed and well-informed. If you are in distress from your condition, consider bringing a friend or family member for support. Counselors and social workers can also serve as health advocates. If you feel your provider is unduly negative about novel treatment options, consider a second opinion.

READ IN CASE OF PUSHBACK

We get emotionally invested in a belief or a viewpoint, and it's hard to see beyond it. Consider the disaster this poses in the world of medicine. Patients suffer unnecessarily when old ideas are irrationally kept alive.

When physicians and patients meet, it's most productive when both parties are prepared. The doctor is supposed to bring her expertise (and knowledge of your case and condition). The patient should bring his questions and concerns.

Keep in mind that your doctor deals with

- overconfident Googlers with a medical degree from last night's browsing. It's hard to treat patients like these because they may have a false sense of expertise, having bathed themselves in information, but perhaps with the inability to draw accurate conclusions.
- passive patients. Sometimes they are passive because they are too ill to fight for themselves. They take whatever the doctor hands them. Others are passive because they don't have the education to ask the right questions. When I shadowed physicians for my graduate work, I noticed a growing divide between patients with medical knowledge and those without.

Of course, when medical appointments are squished into tiny 15-minute blocks, it's almost impossible to address either of these groups.

The main thing is that preparation on your part will pay dividends. FindKetamine.com and the book in your hands are two great places to get your "Ketamine education."

HOW TO OVERCOME OBJECTIONS TO TREATMENT

Even with the positive buzz around low-dose IV Ketamine therapy, some physicians may be skeptical. Talking about Ketamine treatments with a person who is not open to new treatments can be discouraging. You may need a second opinion. Here are a few points to keep in mind.

- There can be a tendency to dismiss innovative therapies outside of the mainstream.
- The medical world is bursting with discovery. No one doctor can keep up with the volume of new developments each day. Many well-educated and experienced physicians may not know about low-dose IV Ketamine.
- It is common for people, including physicians, to only know of Ketamine as an illegal, recreational drug.

But does simply not being educated about Ketamine make it illegitimate? Of course not!

Below are points that might come up during your consultations.

Isn't Ketamine a "Club Drug?"

One of the recreational names for Ketamine is "Special K." Some people use it in a dangerous, recreational environment. In the medical setting, Ketamine's dissociative properties are essential to medical operations worldwide.

Like any drug, it can be abused. But just because a drug can be abused doesn't mean it can't be medically useful.

Is Ketamine FDA Approved?

Whether Ketamine and Esketamine are FDA approved is a common question.

Ketamine

Ketamine was approved for use in the 1960s as an anesthetic. As of 2021, Ketamine's applications span behavioral health, pain conditions, and even treating substance abuse and addiction.

How can Ketamine be used in nonanesthetic settings?

When Ketamine is prescribed for something other than anesthesia, it is being used "off-label." Low-dose IV Ketamine infusions are off-label treatments for a variety of the illnesses mentioned, including depression. Off-label use is legal. However, these "unofficial" applications may make insurance reimbursement less likely. Insurance companies often categorize off-label uses of treatments as "experimental" and not warranting coverage.

One reason off-label permissions are important is that a medication's additional benefits may be noticed years before being officially approved for that purpose. Ketamine, in particular, benefits from off-label use as many of its effects on mental, physical, and addiction-related illnesses emerged incidentally to its prescribed purpose as an anesthetic.

Esketamine

Esketamine is the "mirror" molecule of Ketamine. Patented in 2019, Esketamine (brand name Spravato™) is, unlike Ketamine, specifically FDA approved for relieving treatment-resistant depression.

Esketamine is inhaled through the nose. Its ease of administration, combined with insurance coverage, may expand access to this vital treatment.

No One Knows Everything

Doctors have spent countless hours learning about these diseases and how to treat them. Most care a lot for their patients and want nothing more than to help them.

But does any of this mean that medical professionals are all-knowing? Is it at all possible for there to be another medicine, another herb, another substance, another approach out there that could help?

No one can know everything there is to know about every topic. And it's not a shame to say so. Only when we admit to not knowing everything can we stay open-minded to learning something new. One of the most outstanding qualities in a doctor is not merely knowing something but admitting when they don't.

Keep in mind that the latest treatments are usually practiced by a handful of experienced specialists. Those are the people you need to find.

Your current status doesn't have to be your fate. Consult other doctors offering new options. That testimonial you read online in the middle of the night while you Googled away in desperation, from someone you don't know, from a place you've never heard of, about an unknown drug, could be your ticket out of misery.

Low-dose IV Ketamine therapy is just one possibility. There are many others.

WILL IT WORK FOR ME?

I understand.

THIS is the million-dollar question. THE most important question.

Frank, is it worth it!? Will it help me?

After all, if Ketamine isn't able to help you, why even read one more page?

The truth is, your question has no simple or guaranteed answer.

There are theories about Ketamine's mechanisms and why it may work to alleviate particular symptoms in the short or long term. However, no one knows how Ketamine, or any drug, will affect you as an individual until you consume it. Every medication, particularly psychiatric ones, can make someone feel better, worse, or anywhere in between.

There can be a million studies and promising statistics. The drug could've even worked miraculously for a family member or friend. Still, nothing guarantees its effects on you. Be sure to work closely with your physician and honestly report what you are experiencing.

MAKING THE MOST OUT OF TREATMENT

I want to share what my personal Ketamine doctor (Dr. Henry Macler) told me from the beginning.

(paraphrasing)

Me: How long before this "takes effect?"
Dr. Macler: We find that function often *precedes* feeling.

Not what I wanted to hear.

When you're suffering and in pain, "take effect" means feeling better. I mean, what else matters?? I'm feeling terrible!

But, taking effect can also mean functioning better. How you feel and function can be very different, especially at first. Don't despair! Functioning better can lead to feeling better, especially if you take action.

What my doctor told me is a critical key to success. Take action right away. Make use of your newfound functionality. Do as much as you can. Push your boundaries.

For some people, that's just stepping outside of their homes.

For others, it may be trying out part-time jobs. There are all kinds of big and small steps. Just take steps.

Let me stress this again: don't wait to feel better before you act better.

Why? Three reasons:

1. Ketamine facilitates incremental growth. If you need low-dose IV Ketamine therapy, you have probably fallen behind in life. You won't regain all of that ground overnight. It doesn't matter. The incremental steps are all you need to move forward.
2. The more you accomplish each day, week, or month, the more confidence you'll gain.
3. When you are doing more, your self-image is re-conceptualized. Your sense of self-esteem grows. Your capabilities expand. People around you notice you're emerging from the shadows of dysfunction.

One of the best predictors of treatment success is one's determination to follow through on these principles. Ketamine can provide a unique opportunity to reoccupy your life in new and exciting ways. Decide that you're going to make progress, however little, from day one. There will be steps forward and back. That's OK. That's normal.

Of course, you still need other ways of gauging your success. A later section of the book talks more about how to evaluate your progress.

When you're ready to consult with a doctor or visit a Ketamine clinic, please read the next chapter.

HOW TO FIND A GOOD KETAMINE CLINIC

T he best way to find the right Ketamine clinic is by searching our Ketamine Clinic Directory at <u>FindKetamine.com</u>.

KEY QUESTIONS FOR YOUR DOCTOR

Consulting with your potential Ketamine doctor can be encouraging. I recommend bringing a list of questions to make your exchange easy and productive.

Is this likely to help me?
What is your success rate with cases like mine?
Who will perform my procedure?
What safety measures are in place?
What should I expect?
What are the costs and payment options?
How long is the waiting list for treatment?

It's natural to feel awkward when asking for this type of information. But don't worry. These are reasonable questions in any medical setting.

KEEP YOUR EYES PEELED

During your search for a suitable Ketamine clinic, keep watch for red flags:

Guaranteed Results

In life, there are no guarantees. Ketamine treatments are no exception. Be wary of clinics proclaiming guaranteed results.

Unsupported Claims

Medical statements (called "claims") require evidence. As you walk through your research steps, pay attention to where the information comes from. Does it come from established news outlets or formal medical journals? Does it sound good but has no citations or footnotes supporting it? Of course, one should consider the clinic's ratings and testimonials. But don't let subjective input overwhelm that from more objective sources.

A Dangerous Time for Bargain Shopping

Low-dose IV Ketamine treatment is expensive. One treatment can range from $250-$800 or more, depending on the clinic and the treatment protocol's specifics. With this much money on the line, bargain hunting is tempting, particularly if your income is interrupted by your health status.

But, let me say this: I didn't go with the cheapest clinic. Here's why:

Whenever I can, I try to avoid skimping on healthcare. My health conditions, disability time off from work, and treatment fees have already cost me a fortune. Now I try to work with the best people to get the best results the first time.

Also, I understand that the service and facilities I'm paying for are costly. Ketamine itself is available in generic form and inexpensive. It's the procedural overhead that creates the costs. Staff, liability insurance, office space, and medical equipment are all expensive.

Sure, some clinics will go cheap on these. There are many ways to cut corners. They may buy uncomfortable chairs for the infusion patients. Climate control could be poor within treatment rooms, leaving it either boiling or freezing. They may save on rent, leasing questionable space on the edge of town with no parking. They may also hire staff with less training, education, and experience.

Running a high-quality clinic is deceptively expensive. Keep this in mind during your search.

WHAT IS THE CLINIC'S MOTIVATION?

The relationship between medicine and money is fraught.

On the one hand is the desire to provide medical care to everyone, regardless of their financial status. On the other hand, medicine is also a business. The cost of education, facilities, supplies, insurance, and payroll are real.

When I look for a medical service provider, I try to find someone who cares. Who knows their stuff but is also concerned with my personal case. When a medical business is solely about the money, my concern is whether the patients are receiving the highest quality treatment.

As someone with a background in both business and medicine, I have nothing against the business of medicine. It's right that people profit fairly from their labor. In our economic system, the exchange of money for goods and services is how things work. However, I still look for the signs of caring commitment and reasonable value.

One Doctor's Commitment

Due to all that I've been through health-wise, I am particular about my medical care. Once I decided I wanted to try low-dose IV Ketamine therapy, I needed to find a great clinic headed by a doctor I could trust. When I started searching, I found the contact information for a clinic in the Pittsburgh area directed by Dr. Henry Macler. I looked him up.

He has excellent academic and career credentials. Most importantly, he is an anesthesiologist with an extraordinary amount of experience with Ketamine, including the low-dose IV Ketamine treatments I was seeking out. In fact, it was his long-time colleague and low-dose IV Ketamine treatment pioneer, Dr. Glen Z. Brooks, that convinced him of the therapeutic power of IV Ketamine. Dr. Brooks is well-known as the physician who opened one of the first low-dose IV Ketamine clinics in the US, treating over 4,000 patients.

So far, so good.

But, bouncing around the medical system has taught me something: a doctor's resume doesn't tell you everything about their care.

Caring AND Credentials

Amazingly, I found BOTH in Dr. Macler: 1) his genuine compassion for helping patients and 2) the academic pedigree with an admirable track record of Ketamine administration.

Dr. Macler almost lost his daughter to depression. During our first meeting, he explained how the near tragedy affected his commitment to preventing similar losses. He expressed a genuine depth of concern for his patients and the determination to provide them with safe, effective treatment. Having a doctor who cares, who you feel wants the best for you, can be as important as the best credentials.

But, let's back up. How did I come to have this consultation?

Poor "Doc"

True to my word, I did what I'm recommending to you: I sent him an email, introduced myself, and shared my interest in low-dose IV Ketamine therapy.

He and his ever-patient wife replied the next day. They were probably sorry they did because I started with a mountain of questions. Are you surprised that someone who writes a whole book about Ketamine has a LOT of questions?!

Keep in mind that I'm not good at writing SHORT emails. Something that most people capture in one line takes me ten.

My research advisor in medical school, Dr. Steven Handler, a genuine credit to his profession, told me straight out that he didn't have time to read all my emails. To paraphrase: "Frank, you write beautiful emails. And, if I had the time to kick back with a cup of tea and read them through, I'd probably enjoy them. But I don't have that time. I only sleep a few hours a day as it is!"

Yeah, I felt a bit embarrassed. The real reason my emails are so long is that the OCD makes it nearly impossible for me to finish. A panic comes over me about what I may be missing or not explaining in enough detail. Then, I worry about the tone of the writing. Does it sound respectful? Informed? Well-prepared? I'm typing and typing, and before I know it, I'm totally stressed out from reading and rereading. In the end, in a world of sound bytes and texts, I produce this encyclopedia of an email just to ask if you think something's a good idea.

Back to poor Dr. Macler. My questions kept pouring in. Mind you, he's already running a busy Ketamine clinic, conferring with colleagues, and consulting with patients. Then some guy comes equipped with a deluge of questions, many of which do not have a quick yes or no answer. But there I was, just going all-in on this interrogation, drawing on his expertise, experiences, and opinions. I had already spent over a year investigating low-dose IV Ketamine treatments. As an educated consumer, I was not only trying to understand more about Ketamine but also evaluate him as my potential provider.

To the good doctor's credit and translated through his wife Jean's wisdom, the humbly knowledgeable answers kept coming. Eventually, they politely suggested that I call or come in for a consult. Who can blame them? I sounded like I'd go on forever!

Once again, I felt a bit embarrassed. I often feel like I'm asking too much of someone and don't want to get rejected. But asking me to spend some focused time getting my questions answered to make a decision was certainly reasonable.

Finally, meeting Dr. Macler in person, I joyfully discovered a kind, thoughtful, and experienced practitioner. His sincere nature conveyed through our earlier emails matched his demeanor.

The Real Dope

Dr. Macler never hyped up the potential results. He never tried to sell me on Ketamine. He didn't pretend to know if or when I would feel better. Sure, he shared the statistics that encouraged his practice, but he was the first to admit that many questions about low-dose IV Ketamine therapy remain unanswered. I give him tremendous credit for his integrity in balancing the business of medicine.

He also gave me the "bad news" about patients often "doing better" before they are "feeling better." This phenomenon of functional improvements manifesting before mood-based benefits is common in Ketamine treatment. I'm glad he shared this fact upfront. It tempered my expectations. Knowing the importance of "acting better" before I "felt better" set me up for long-term success.

Adding all of this up, my face-to-face consultation with Dr. Macler, his wife, and the medical team sealed the deal. I knew this was the place for me. I knew I'd be safe and surrounded by people who cared about me and my future.

This clinic, the Pittsburgh branch of one of the nation's first IV Ketamine clinics (New York Ketamine Infusions, headed by Dr. Glen Brooks), is very experienced with thousands of treatments under its belt.

And they see results.

A WORD ABOUT EXPECTATIONS

Low-dose IV Ketamine does a lot for me. But I always tell people what my doctor told me: keep realistic expectations. When we are ill, we seek relief. The ideal relief is a cure, of course. But relief is a good runner-up.

Why do I bring this up?

Because when I go for my Ketamine infusions, I know they are a source of relief. When I'm having a brutal stretch of bipolar depression or OCD, Ketamine helps clear my mind and recharges me emotionally to get back up and try again. Still, I don't go into a treatment expecting to throw all of my medications into the trash on my way out.

THE KETAMINE EXPERIENCE

Perhaps the most popular question: what do Ketamine infusions feel like? Are they frightening? Do you feel out of control?

Being "high" on Ketamine or on a Ketamine "trip" is a unique and difficult-to-articulate experience. I'll go into detail below.

Before that, here are tips for making your Ketamine treatments relaxing, enjoyable, and therapeutic.

SET AND SETTING ARE KEY!

When you're first starting out in Ketamine therapy, you can make the most out of your experiences by attending to your "set" and "setting." It is only when I've violated these points that my "trip" was unpleasant.

"Set" refers to one's mindset. The "setting" refers to the treatment environment.

Preparing Your Mindset

It may seem unreasonable to extol the virtues of "feeling good mentally" to patients like us who, by definition, are there because we do NOT feel good! A more reasonable goal is to position yourself as well as possible for the experience.

What does this include?

- **Rest.** I've found that heading into a Ketamine treatment without the proper rest can increase discomfort. When you are rested, the body is calm (as it can be). Keep in mind that any change, even when positive, is stressful to the system. So, one should try to be "firing on all cylinders" going in. Also, I've found that a lack of sleep draws on the adrenals and can lead to adrenaline-induced anxiety or uncomfortable fluctuations in blood sugar levels.

- **Mental hygiene.** We all have a lot on our minds. It could be what happened last night or the fear that we will never recover from our current hell. Again, one can only do one's best to keep things as mentally uncluttered as possible. Avoid arguments, over-stimulating TV or music, news, and even conversations with friends or family that upset you. You can always pick these back up later if you want. But minimize them going in.

- **Food.** Your doctor will provide instructions for your eating schedule. You will be required to abstain from eating a certain number of hours before treatment. Keep the digestive system regular and working properly. Not following your doctor's instructions is a safety hazard. Ketamine, like any anesthetic, should only be administered on an empty stomach to prevent serious complications.

- **One more note about food.** In the day or two leading up to your treatment, stick to foods your system digests well. This isn't the time to try that new spicy Indian dish or stay up late eating greasy pizza. During one of my treatments, I was experiencing indigestion from a meal the night before. It decreased the quality of the Ketamine experience, as I felt the pain and heaviness of my stomach all the way through.

- **Medications.** Your doctor will provide instructions for how to handle your medications. She may ask you to adjust your regimen prior to the treatment. Follow these instructions for your safety and for the best treatment outcome. For instance, some drugs such as Benzodiazepines may interfere with Ketamine's action. Your doctor may have you reduce or delay a dose leading up to your Ketamine treatment.

- **Meditation.** Meditation does not have to be formal. It can be prayer, daydreaming, or just giving yourself time off from trying to think about everything going on in your life. It's good to "meditate" leading up to your treatment. Anything that keeps your mind at peace and open to surrender is positive.

What Makes a Good Setting?

Experienced low-dose IV Ketamine practitioners understand the critical importance of their treatment environment. That environment is composed of everything beginning with how one is greeted all the way through the conclusion of the treatment and one's exit. Consider these factors.

- The "vibe" or culture of the clinic is key. Patients coming in with severe mental and physical illness are already under stress. They need to be cared for, treated kindly, and with patience.

- The surroundings should be quiet and comfortable. Suitable furniture, temperature, and beverages reinforce a sense of tranquility and safety.

- The doctor needs to spend time with the patient to understand their unique case and concerns. Having a Ketamine treatment comes with questions. A caring doctor addresses everything the patient asks and provides reassurance.

- The staff that administers the actual treatment is also very important. Considerations for the comfortable placement of the IV, orientation of the treatment chair, and monitoring of the patient's vitals are all important.

Because you will be interacting mostly with this staff, it's helpful when they have a kind, soothing demeanor.

- During the Ketamine treatment itself, the patient's environment needs protection from unnecessary sensory stimuli, including uncomfortable heat or cold, bright lights, stressful or startling noises, and unwanted company (some patients prefer to undergo treatment without anyone else in the room and minimal checkups by the staff).

- Coming out from under the influence of Ketamine should be gradual and unhurried. One will feel groggy and disoriented. This isn't necessarily an unpleasant experience. A great treatment session is pleasurable during and after. Personally, I feel very good and relaxed for the rest of the day. A calm environment will help facilitate a smooth transition back into full awareness.

- Post-treatment time should include the ability to relax on comfortable furniture or be driven home in a nurturing and serene environment. You will likely feel a sense of joy and freedom. Prolong it by planning your logistics ahead of time.

- When you are ready, along with the caretaker accompanying you, the same conditions that provide a comfortable, uneventful transition back into normal consciousness should be maintained as long as possible.

STEP-BY-STEP OF THE INFUSION PROCEDURE

Arrive at the office early for paperwork. You may be asked to fill out questionnaires regarding the status and severity of your health condition.

Usually, you pay upfront. (While you can still remember where your wallet is!)

You'll be ushered into a treatment room. Usually, these have reclining chairs, relative quiet, and dimmable lights. You sit down and get comfortable. Discussions about the dose are finalized before the Ketamine is prepared.

Commonly, small doses of the anti-nausea medication Zofran are supplied prior to treatment. This prevents the effects of disorientation from becoming nauseating.

Upon your arm is placed a blood pressure cuff and a pulse oximeter. During a low-dose IV Ketamine infusion, your vital signs are monitored, including your EKG, pulse, and oxygen levels.

The nurse inserts the IV via a small needle, usually in the hand. Once the IV is secure, the liquid bag of Ketamine is hung, and administration into your bloodstream begins. You will soon feel relaxed.

The staff will check on you at regular intervals to make sure you are not experiencing discomfort. Some clinics have protocols like pushing a button or making a thumbs down sign in case of distress.

Now, just kick back and enjoy!

What is it Like?

Everyone experiences Ketamine differently, so I'll share my own journey.

First, I feel a wave of relaxation and knowing that I'm safe from the world. Then, I feel a warm, joy building from the bottom chakra up through my body. I can still think and direct my thoughts; they just aren't so "sticky." I'm free of obsession and can watch my thoughts more clearly.

Ketamine affects proprioception, one's sense of orientation in space. Even though I'm sitting upright in the chair, it feels like it's reclining into a flat position. I know I'm not moving physically, nor is the chair. But the sensations of moving are as convincing as in real life. But I don't feel nauseous. I still feel calm and curious. If anything, the repositioning of my body in space is calming.

This reorientation in space continues until my chair has slowly rotated me completely upside down. The floor is now above me, and all of the room's furniture is now appropriately rearranged to reflect this new perspective.

I'm a big fan of having my treatments in sensory-deprived environments. Sounds are blocked out by my headphones, lights are turned off, sunglasses are on, and eyes are closed. Vibrant shapes emerge. Not random or tree-like or like lightning or everyday objects. They're geometric objects like rectangles and unfolding doors. Traces of their movement leave brief trails of light.

Music

Of all the types of music I've listened to under Ketamine, opera is my favorite. Why? Well, I do like opera even while sober. But, more importantly, the music slows down in my mind. Each syllable becomes close and intimate. The vocalist is no longer a stranger on a distant stage. Rather, I'm a friend, tremendously moved by their performance and standing very close by.

People

One thing I never "see" is people, not people I know nor others. Nor do I see any kind of "movie." But, some patients do.

Awakening

You will likely wake slowly. You may have gone fully to sleep or just into a twilight state.

Take your time getting up. Be safe. You may be surprised at your level of intoxication.

Begin rehydrating yourself and using the restroom. Ketamine has a diuretic effect.

Is Ketamine Therapy a Good Experience?

Yes, *low-dose IV Ketamine treatment can be an amazing experience.*

Many factors influence one's Ketamine infusion experience. My list of tips above will increase your chances of a pleasant journey.

One's experience with surrendering to dissociative states may impact the characterization of their treatment. I can't back up this supposition with real data. This is just something I've noticed in talking with doctors and patients.

For instance, patients who have experience with drug or alcohol use might be less likely to "freak out" during the Ketamine "trip." They relax into the sensations more quickly and are more comfortable letting go of control. Patients with a tendency towards maintaining strict control of their inner world may find the loosening of their grip disturbing or stressful. Either way, you will only be under the dissociative influence of the Ketamine for an hour or two.

The good news is: You need not worry about how you feel during the treatment. It's my opinion that whether the "trip" is delightful or hair-raising, the healing benefits still take place. I've had "great" trips and anxious ones, and my progress continued unabated.

K-holes and When Things Go "Wrong"

Ketamine infusions are great fun for some and frightening for others. Speaking for myself, Ketamine doesn't increase my anxiety (except during a bad K-hole). During therapy, I find obsessive and anxious thoughts temporarily vanish.

Then again, everyone is different, and I've had a lot of experience by now. Just know it's OK to experience anxiety before, during, or after treatment.

Bad Trips and K-holes: What are they?

Ketamine can induce a "bad trip" or "K-hole."

K-holes do not have a formal definition. It's a general term to describe a Ketamine experience that is uncomfortable, frightening, or feels dangerous. For instance, one may consider having been in a K-hole when their Ketamine session involved anxiety, terror, or hallucinations. These effects can result from Ketamine's dissociative properties..

Being in a K-hole usually denotes extreme versions of the effects below.

- Confusion
- Slurred and difficult to articulate speech
- Subjective experiences that are hard to communicate
- Sensations of flying or floating
- "Out of body" experiences

- Mystical or transcendent experiences that may be categorized as near-death, astral, or religious
- Paranoia about not being able to "wake up" from the disassociation

It's important to note that many descriptions of bad experiences with Ketamine are connected to recreational use and higher doses than those given during a low-dose IV Ketamine treatment. Recreational Ketamine users may ingest many times the dose of that administered during prescribed Ketamine therapy. They also do so under vastly different circumstances than those offered by a clinic. These factors make K-hole experiences much more likely and potentially frightening.

Unfortunately, disturbing critiques of low-dose Ketamine therapy are often confused with those of recreational use. There is a big difference.

The most intensely frightening experience in K-holes varies between patients. One theme with which I'm personally familiar is a form of being buried alive.

6 Feet Down

The room and the reality within somehow slowed down. Even though I couldn't visually identify anything and nothing obvious had changed, I just "knew" the molecules of reality were slowing to an unnatural stop.

During this time, I was in a continually more confined space. Ketamine causes paralysis at higher doses (one reason it's good for anesthesia). But, in this K-hole, the inability to move, combined with the sense of being buried deep underground, was terrifying. My breathing felt (but wasn't) constricted. Everything was dark, and this deep grave was inescapable. All movement down to the quantum world had stopped. There was nothing except eternal stillness.

It was scary. But, before long, I was ascending from my tomb and able to move and breathe normally.

So yes, it is possible to have an anxiety-provoking experience. But that has only happened to me a few times out of many. The dose was too high, and I probably didn't follow the tips I'm giving you.

Even when a therapy session is scary, it can change the way you perceive your life and reality in general. You get to explore this other world to which you usually don't have access. Low-dose IV Ketamine can be a true revelation inaccessible in daily life.

No matter what is going on. Don't worry! Even if you're uncomfortable, it'll be over soon. Ketamine wears off quickly. The psychological journeys tend to end immediately upon the cessation of the infusion. If, on the other hand, you're celebrating the "ride," you'll be disappointed it's over so soon!

DO "BAD TRIPS" IMPEDE TREATMENT?

Even when you have a trying experience, the effect of the treatment may still be as useful as that following a "good trip." In other words, my sense is that even a hair-raising session does not necessarily indicate what the long-term result will be. Bad trip ≠ bad results.

Some patients drop out of low-dose IV Ketamine treatments due to uncomfortable experiences. This can be because of the experience itself. But it can also be because of the unknown relationship between those couple hours of experience and the long-term results of the treatment.

My philosophy is to only consider a "bad trip" one where BOTH the experience is unpleasant AND lacks therapeutic benefit in the short or long term.

KETAMINE AND PSYCHOLOGICAL THERAPY

Consider the example of someone who, under the influence of Ketamine, revisits a traumatic experience from their past. Sometimes, people in that situation are able to "watch" or "observe" the trauma from a disassociated distance, not reliving the pain of the trauma, *per se*, but rather viewing it in a new light. However, there are also cases when one re-experiences the pain of the trauma.

There are therapists who specialize in working with patients undergoing low-dose IV Ketamine treatment. This combined approach is usually referred to as either Ketamine Assisted Therapy (KAT) or Ketamine Psychedelic Therapy (KPT).

Adjunct psychological therapy may yield additional benefits, such as the ability to let go of deeply ingrained emotions and thought patterns more easily. This is an additional level of intervention that I would like to try myself.

RESULTS

People often ask me how I feel and if low-dose IV Ketamine has made a difference in my life. When you've had a long-term serious health problem, it can be hard to judge or even remember what is "normal." With so much time spent living on the edge, how can you evaluate whether you've really made it back?

Knowing what relief means to you will help you gauge your results more honestly.

WHAT'S YOUR PERSONAL DEFINITION OF RELIEF?

Now, when we define "alleviate" or "relief," it's all a matter of degrees. In clinical settings, standardized tests or "inventories" are used to quantify a patient's severity of anxiety or depression. For instance, let's say a patient begins with an "8" on some scale of depression. Alleviation may be as minor as a reduction to "7" or as dramatic as a reduction to "0."

Will I Feel Better?

Clinical data, as well as feedback I've personally received from doctors experienced with Ketamine treatment, suggest that low-dose IV Ketamine's track record concerning treatment-resistant depression shows that approximately *two-thirds* of patients experience significant improvement.

This rate of success usually applies to an approach to Ketamine treatment which includes six treatments within 2–3 weeks. Some patients begin feeling better within their first treatment. Some not until later treatments. Some don't seem to respond at all.

Ketamine doesn't work for everyone. However, the percentage of patients that it does help is astounding, particularly in such a brief period of treatment. Standard psychiatric medications take 2-12 weeks to work.

HOW DO YOU EVALUATE YOUR RESULTS?

Below is the framework I use to monitor progress.

Internal: Do I feel better? Have my symptoms lessened? Can I work or carry out my responsibilities more successfully and consistently? Am I getting closer to reaching my goals?

External: What are my family and friends saying? Am I acting better or worse? Is my behavior changing for the better?

Professional: What do my therapist and psychiatrist think? Do they see emotional or functional progress from my treatments?

Please don't ignore these perspectives because it's easy to FEEL like we're not doing better, even when other people are sure that we ARE. When we can't see our situation from all sides, we make unbalanced assessments and poor decisions. When you combine these three viewpoints, you'll have a clearer picture of your progress.

MY KETAMINE REPORT CARD

After two years of treatment, here's my truth: *Yes, it has definitely helped my depression.*

Suicidal thoughts were my constant companion. They NEVER let up. It was a never-ending, one-sided conversation: "I can't take this pain anymore. It will never stop. What else can I do? I'm not living. I'm not even getting by. I'm in agony."

Now, those haunting thoughts are virtually gone. They've been gone since early in my treatments. The relief from that eternal sense of impending destruction, combined with the determination to make progress, is what has brought me this far.

Why does relief from suicidal thoughts mean so much?

For many years, my mind kept saying, "This is too overwhelming. I can't get a moment of peace. What if something else happens on top of this? I'll just crumble. I'm out of reserves. I'm just in shambles." This soundtrack intensifies the depression that initially brought them on. It's a circle. Feeling helpless. Feeling hopeless. Both of these drive you deeper into the pit.

THE RECOVERY CONTINUES

My experience has been positive so far. I know to expect improvements in functionality to precede "feeling better." I find it's helpful to push my boundaries, even before I "feel" like it because the Ketamine supports me.

Ketamine may continually act upon the brain, nervous system, or other aspects of the body for unknown lengths of time. From what I've learned and experienced, I do believe that Ketamine continues to exert its effects upon my brain long after the treatment itself. Even though Ketamine is metabolized quickly in the body, long-term or cumulative effects may still be discovered.

THE BOTTOM LINE

After undergoing more than two years of treatments, I can report that low dose IV Ketamine is *very effective for my treatment-resistant depression*. It has made a tremendous difference in my life. And after decades of suffering, I'm very thankful to have found it.

Has low-dose IV Ketamine helped me? **Absolutely.**

Will I continue with more treatments as needed? **Absolutely.**

Do I hope that more sufferers hear about Ketamine? **Absolutely.**

HOW MANY TREATMENTS DO I NEED?

The most common regimen for Ketamine infusions is to begin with a rapid sequence of infusions over the first few weeks. After that, practitioners may differ concerning the going-forward therapy plan.

I'm fortunate in that my suicidal ideations began lessening within my first and second infusion treatments. Those thoughts stay at bay as I receive a Ketamine treatment once a month.

Speaking for myself and from what I've seen, when one does feel better, relief may or may not persist. Periodic boosters may be required.

The only way to know with certainty what your results and treatment needs will be is to undergo treatment yourself. As each person is different, so is their treatment plan.

NEXT STEPS

Thank you for purchasing this book. Please share it with family and friends.

Spread the news about Ketamine, a *new hope for patients with difficult-to-treat illnesses.*

FindKetamine.com contains all of the resources you need to move forward. Our directory of Ketamine clinics will help you find the right place.

Subscribe to our newsletter for tips and strategies to help you navigate this life-changing treatment. Also, get exclusive access to little-known payment strategies to afford the treatments you need.

Would you rather discuss these topics one on one? Please book a call with "The Ketamine Coach," Frank M. Ligons at FindKetamine.com.

Did you enjoy this book? Do you feel more hopeful?

I hope so!

If you feel my book is worthwhile, please
don't forget to leave an honest review.

Every review matters, and it matters a lot!

Your review can be submitted through
Amazon or your bookseller.

I thank you endlessly!

Are you considering Ketamine?

Would you like to know more?

Please visit us at <u>FindKetamine.com</u>

SELECTED BIBLIOGRAPHY

aan het Rot, M., Collins, K. A., Murrough, J. W., Perez, A. M., Reich, D. L., Charney, D. S., & Mathew, S. J. (2010). Safety and efficacy of repeated-dose intravenous ketamine for treatment-resistant depression. *Biological Psychiatry, 67*(2), 139–145. https://doi.org/10.1016/j.biopsych.2009.08.038

Acevedo-Diaz, E. E., Cavanaugh, G. W., Greenstein, D., Kraus, C., Kadriu, B., Zarate, C. A., & Park, L. T. (2020). Comprehensive assessment of side effects associated with a single dose of ketamine in treatment-resistant depression. *Journal of Affective Disorders, 263*, 568–575. https://doi.org/10.1016/j.jad.2019.11.028

Adachi, M., Barrot, M., Autry, A. E., Theobald, D., & Monteggia, L. M. (2008). Selective loss of bdnf in the dentate gyrus attenuates antidepressant efficacy. *Biological Psychiatry, 63*(7), 642–649. https://doi.org/10.1016/j.biopsych.2007.09.019

Addiction support groups. (n.d.). Addiction Center. Retrieved March 22, 2021, from https://www.addictioncenter.com/treatment/support-groups/

Berman, R. M., Cappiello, A., Anand, A., Oren, D. A., Heninger, G. R., Charney, D. S., & Krystal, J. H. (2000). Antidepressant effects of ketamine in depressed patients. *Biological Psychiatry, 47*(4), 351–354. https://doi.org/10.1016/s0006-3223(99)00230-9

Beurel, E., Song, L., & Jope, R. S. (2011). Inhibition of glycogen synthase kinase-3 is necessary for the rapid antidepressant effect of ketamine in mice. *Molecular Psychiatry, 16*(11), 1068–1070. https://doi.org/10.1038/mp.2011.47

Björkholm, C., & Monteggia, L. M. (2016). BDNF - a key transducer of antidepressant effects. *Neuropharmacology, 102*, 72–79. https://doi.org/10.1016/j.neuropharm.2015.10.034

Bloch, M. H., Wasylink, S., Landeros-Weisenberger, A., Panza, K. E., Billingslea, E., Leckman, J. F., Krystal, J. H., Bhagwagar, Z., Sanacora, G., & Pittenger, C. (2012). Effects of ketamine in treatment-refractory obsessive-compulsive disorder. *Biological Psychiatry, 72*(11), 964–970. https://doi.org/10.1016/j.biopsych.2012.05.028

Cohen, S. P., Bhatia, A., Buvanendran, A., Schwenk, E. S., Wasan, A. D., Hurley, R. W., Viscusi, E. R., Narouze, S., Davis, F. N., Ritchie, E. C., Lubenow, T. R., & Hooten, W. M. (2018). Consensus guidelines on the use of intravenous ketamine infusions for chronic pain from the american society of regional anesthesia and pain medicine, the american academy of pain medicine, and the american society of anesthesiologists. *Regional Anesthesia and Pain Medicine, 43*(5), 521–546. https://doi.org/10.1097/AAP.0000000000000808

Connery, H. S. (2015). Medication-assisted treatment of opioid use disorder: Review of the evidence and future directions. *Harvard Review of Psychiatry, 23*(2), 63–75. https://doi.org/10.1097/HRP.0000000000000075

Corriger, A., & Pickering, G. (2019). Ketamine and depression: A narrative review. *Drug Design, Development and Therapy, 13*, 3051–3067. https://doi.org/10.2147/DDDT.S221437

D'Andrea, D., & Sewell, R. A. (2013). Transient resolution of treatment-resistant posttraumatic stress disorder following ketamine infusion. *Biological Psychiatry, 74*(9), e13–e14. https://doi.org/10.1016/j.biopsych.2013.04.019

December 9, E. S. U. & 2019. (n.d.-a). *Physical symptoms of ketamine abuse: Short-term & physiological effects*. American Addiction Centers. Retrieved March 22, 2021, from https://americanaddictioncenters.org/ketamine-abuse/physical-symptoms

December 9, E. S. U. & 2019. (n.d.-b). *The side effects of ketamine—Treatment options*. American Addiction Centers. Retrieved March 22, 2021, from https://americanaddictioncenters.org/ketamine-abuse/ketamine-side-effects

DiazGranados, N., Ibrahim, L. A., Brutsche, N. E., Ameli, R., Henter, I. D., Luckenbaugh, D. A., Machado-Vieira, R., & Zarate, C. A. (2010). Rapid resolution of suicidal ideation after a single infusion of an N-methyl-D-aspartate antagonist in patients with treatment-resistant major depressive disorder. *The Journal of Clinical Psychiatry*, *71*(12), 1605–1611. https://doi.org/10.4088/JCP.09m05327blu

Disorders, I. of M. (US) F. on N. and N. S. (2011). *Overview of the glutamatergic system*. National Academies Press (US). https://www.ncbi.nlm.nih.gov/books/NBK62187/

Domino, E. F., & Warner, D. S. (2010). Taming the ketamine tiger. *Anesthesiology*, *113*(3), 678–684. https://doi.org/10.1097/ALN.0b013e3181ed09a2

Donoghue, A. C., Roback, M. G., & Cullen, K. R. (2015). Remission from behavioral dysregulation in a child with ptsd after receiving procedural ketamine. *Pediatrics*, *136*(3), e694-696. https://doi.org/10.1542/peds.2014-4152

Europe pmc. (n.d.). Retrieved March 22, 2021, from https://europepmc.org/article/med/23706680

Fda approves esketamine nasal spray for hard-to-treat depression. (n.d.). NPR.Org. Retrieved March 22, 2021, from https://www.npr.org/sections/health-shots/2019/03/05/700509903/fda-clears-esketamine-nasal-spray-for-hard-to-treat-depression

Feder, A., Parides, M. K., Murrough, J. W., Perez, A. M., Morgan, J. E., Saxena, S., Kirkwood, K., aan het Rot, M., Lapidus, K. A. B., Wan, L.-B., Iosifescu, D., & Charney, D. S. (2014). Efficacy of intravenous ketamine for treatment of chronic posttraumatic stress disorder: A randomized clinical trial. *JAMA Psychiatry*, *71*(6), 681. https://doi.org/10.1001/jamapsychiatry.2014.62

Fukumoto, K., Toki, H., Iijima, M., Hashihayata, T., Yamaguchi, J., Hashimoto, K., & Chaki, S. (2017). Antidepressant potential of (R)-

ketamine in rodent models: Comparison with (S)-ketamine. *Journal of Pharmacology and Experimental Therapeutics, 361*(1), 9–16. https://doi.org/10.1124/jpet.116.239228

Gamma-aminobutyric acid (Gaba): Overview, uses, side effects, precautions, interactions, dosing and reviews. (n.d.). Retrieved March 22, 2021, from https://www.webmd.com/vitamins/ai/ingredientmono-464/gamma-aminobutyric-acid-gaba

Hashimoto, K. (2016). Ketamine's antidepressant action: Beyond NMDA receptor inhibition. *Expert Opinion on Therapeutic Targets, 20*(11), 1389–1392. https://doi.org/10.1080/14728222.2016.1238899

Hashimoto, K. (2019). Rapid-acting antidepressant ketamine, its metabolites and other candidates: A historical overview and future perspective. *Psychiatry and Clinical Neurosciences, 73*(10), 613–627. https://doi.org/10. 1/pcn.12902

Hasselmann, H. W. W. (2014). Ketamine as antidepressant? Current state and future perspectives. *Current Neuropharmacology, 12*(1), 57–70. https://doi.org/10.2174/1570159X113119990043

How much does a clinical trial cost? (2020, January 2). *Sofpromed.* https://www.sofpromed.com/how-much-does-a-clinical-trial-cost/

Iv ketamine for adults with mdd or bipolar disorder: Safety and tolerability. (2020, August 10). Psychiatry Advisor. https://www.psychiatryadvisor.com/home/depression-advisor/iv-ketamine-for-adults-with-mdd-or-bipolar-disorder-safety-and-tolerability/

Jesulola, E., Micalos, P., & Baguley, I. J. (2018). Understanding the pathophysiology of depression: From monoamines to the neurogenesis hypothesis model - are we there yet? *Behavioural Brain Research, 341*, 79–90. https://doi.org/10.1016/j.bbr.2017.12.025

Jones, J. L., Mateus, C. F., Malcolm, R. J., Brady, K. T., & Back, S. E. (2018). Efficacy of ketamine in the treatment of substance use disorders:

A systematic review. *Frontiers in Psychiatry, 9.*
https://doi.org/10.3389/fpsyt.2018.00277

Ketalar (Ketamine) dosing, indications, interactions, adverse effects, and more.
(n.d.). Retrieved March 22, 2021, from
https://reference.medscape.com/drug/ketalar-ketamine-343099#3

Ketamine: A promising agent for managing treatment-resistant depression.
(2018, February 19). Psychiatry Advisor.
https://www.psychiatryadvisor.com/home/depression-advisor/ketamine-
a-promising-agent-for-managing-treatment-resistant-depression/

Ketamine: A transformational catalyst. (n.d.-a). MAPS. Retrieved March 22,
2021, from https://maps.org/news/bulletin/articles/410-bulletin-winter-
2016/6470-ketamine-a-transformational-catalyst

Ketamine for depression and mood disorders. (n.d.). *Townsend Letter.*
Retrieved March 22, 2021, from
https://www.townsendletter.com/article/438-ketamine-for-depression-
and-mood-disorders/

Ketamine: Modern drug of abuse? (n.d.-b). Drugs.Com. Retrieved March 22,
2021, from https://www.drugs.com/illicit/ketamine.html

Ketamine research in russia. (n.d.). Retrieved March 22, 2021, from
https://maps.org/research-archive/ketamine/ketrussia.html

Ketamine-assisted therapy. (n.d.). Sage Institute. Retrieved March 22, 2021,
from https://sageinst.org/kat

Klaus, C., Wasserman, D., Henter, I. D., Acevedo-Diaz, E., Kadriu, B., &
Zarate, C. A. (2019). The influence of ketamine on drug discovery in
depression. *Drug Discovery Today, 24*(10), 2033–2043.
https://doi.org/10.1016/j.drudis.2019.07.007

Krupitsky, E. M., & Grinenko, A. Y. (1997). Ketamine psychedelic therapy
(Kpt): A review of the results of ten years of research. *Journal of
Psychoactive Drugs, 29*(2), 165–183.
https://doi.org/10.1080/02791072.1997.10400185

Liriano, F., Hatten, C., & Schwartz, T. L. (2019). Ketamine as treatment for post-traumatic stress disorder: A review. *Drugs in Context, 8.* https://doi.org/10.7573/dic.212305

Lu, Y.-Y., Lin, C.-H., & Lane, H.-Y. (2016). Mania following ketamine abuse. *Neuropsychiatric Disease and Treatment, 12,* 237–239. https://doi.org/10.2147/NDT.S97696

Makin, S. (n.d.). *Behind the buzz: How ketamine changes the depressed patient's brain.* Scientific American. Retrieved March 22, 2021, from https://www.scientificamerican.com/article/behind-the-buzz-how-ketamine-changes-the-depressed-patients-brain/

Matveychuk, D., Thomas, R. K., Swainson, J., Khullar, A., MacKay, M.-A., Baker, G. B., & Dursun, S. M. (2020). Ketamine as an antidepressant: Overview of its mechanisms of action and potential predictive biomarkers. *Therapeutic Advances in Psychopharmacology, 10.* https://doi.org/10.1177/2045125320916657

McGowan, J. C., LaGamma, C. T., Lim, S. C., Tsitsiklis, M., Neria, Y., Brachman, R. A., & Denny, C. A. (2017). Prophylactic ketamine attenuates learned fear. *Neuropsychopharmacology, 42*(8), 1577–1589. https://doi.org/10.1038/npp.2017.19

Moda-Sava, R. N., Murdock, M. H., Parekh, P. K., Fetcho, R. N., Huang, B. S., Huynh, T. N., Witztum, J., Shaver, D. C., Rosenthal, D. L., Alway, E. J., Lopez, K., Meng, Y., Nellissen, L., Grosenick, L., Milner, T. A., Deisseroth, K., Bito, H., Kasai, H., & Liston, C. (2019). Sustained rescue of prefrontal circuit dysfunction by antidepressant-induced spine formation. *Science (New York, N.Y.), 364*(6436). https://doi.org/10.1126/science.aat8078

Newcomer, J. W., Farber, N. B., & Olney, J. W. (2000). NMDA receptor function, memory, and brain aging. *Dialogues in Clinical Neuroscience, 2*(3), 219–232.

Niciu, M. J., Luckenbaugh, D. A., Ionescu, D. F., Richards, E. M., Vande Voort, J. L., Ballard, E. D., Brutsche, N. E., Furey, M. L., & Zarate, C.

A., Jr. (2015). Ketamine's antidepressant efficacy is extended for at least four weeks in subjects with a family history of an alcohol use disorder. *International Journal of Neuropsychopharmacology*, *18*(pyu039). https://doi.org/10.1093/ijnp/pyu039

Nimh » bipolar disorder. (n.d.). Retrieved March 22, 2021, from https://www.nimh.nih.gov/health/statistics/bipolar-disorder.shtml

Nimh » suicide in america: Frequently asked questions. (n.d.). Retrieved March 22, 2021, from https://www.nimh.nih.gov/health/publications/suicide-faq/index.shtml

Pary, R., Matuschka, P. R., Lewis, S., & Lippmann, S. (2006). Managing bipolar depression. *Psychiatry (Edgmont)*, *3*(2), 30–41.

Perez-Caballero, L., Perez, V., & Berrocoso, E. (2020). What ketamine can teach us about the opioid system in depression? *Expert Opinion on Drug Discovery*, *15*(12), 1369–1372. https://doi.org/10.1080/17460441.2020.1781812

Ricke, A. K., Snook, R. J., & Anand, A. (2011). Induction of prolonged mania during ketamine therapy for reflex sympathetic dystrophy. *Biological Psychiatry*, *70*(4), e13-14. https://doi.org/10.1016/j.biopsych.2011.02.030

Rodrigues, N. B., McIntyre, R. S., Lipsitz, O., Lee, Y., Cha, D. S., Nasri, F., Gill, H., Lui, L. M. W., Subramaniapillai, M., Kratiuk, K., Lin, K., Ho, R., Mansur, R. B., & Rosenblat, J. D. (2020). Safety and tolerability of IV ketamine in adults with major depressive or bipolar disorder: Results from the Canadian rapid treatment center of excellence. *Expert Opinion on Drug Safety*, *19*(8), 1031–1040. https://doi.org/10.1080/14740338.2020.1776699

Rodriguez, C. I., Kegeles, L. S., Flood, P., & Simpson, and H. B. (2011). *Rapid resolution of obsessions after an infusion of intravenous ketamine in a patient with treatment-resistant obsessive-compulsive disorder.* 72. https://doi.org/10.4088/JCP.10l06653

Rodriguez, C. I., Kegeles, L. S., Levinson, A., Feng, T., Marcus, S. M., Vermes, D., Flood, P., & Simpson, H. B. (2013). Randomized controlled crossover trial of ketamine in obsessive-compulsive disorder: Proof-of-concept. *Neuropsychopharmacology: Official Publication of the American College of Neuropsychopharmacology*, *38*(12), 2475–2483. https://doi.org/10.1038/npp.2013.150

Rosenbaum, S. B., Gupta, V., & Palacios, J. L. (2021). Ketamine. In *StatPearls*. StatPearls Publishing. http://www.ncbi.nlm.nih.gov/books/NBK470357/

Schizophrenia and aud. (n.d.). Psychiatric Times. Retrieved March 22, 2021, from https://www.psychiatrictimes.com/view/schizophrenia-aud

Schwartz, J., Murrough, J. W., & Iosifescu, D. V. (2016a). Ketamine for treatment-resistant depression: Recent developments and clinical applications. *Evidence-Based Mental Health*, *19*(2), 35–38. https://doi.org/10.1136/eb-2016-102355

Schwartz, J., Murrough, J. W., & Iosifescu, D. V. (2016b). Ketamine for treatment-resistant depression: Recent developments and clinical applications. *Evidence-Based Mental Health*, *19*(2), 35–38. https://doi.org/10.1136/eb-2016-102355

Serafini, G., Howland, R. H., Rovedi, F., Girardi, P., & Amore, M. (2014). The role of ketamine in treatment-resistant depression: A systematic review. *Current Neuropharmacology*, *12*(5), 444–461. https://doi.org/10.2174/1570159X12666140619204251

Shirayama, Y., Chen, A. C.-H., Nakagawa, S., Russell, D. S., & Duman, R. S. (2002). Brain-derived neurotrophic factor produces antidepressant effects in behavioral models of depression. *The Journal of Neuroscience: The Official Journal of the Society for Neuroscience*, *22*(8), 3251–3261. https://doi.org/20026292

Smith-Apeldoorn, S. Y., Veraart, J. K. E., Kamphuis, J., van Asselt, A. D. I., Touw, D. J., aan het Rot, M., & Schoevers, R. A. (2019). Oral esketamine for treatment-resistant depression: Rationale and design of a randomized controlled trial. *BMC Psychiatry*, *19*(1), 375. https://doi.org/10.1186/s12888-019-2359-1

Spravato® (Esketamine) | spravato®. (2020, May 1). SPRAVATO® (Esketamine). https://www.spravato.com/home-1

The ketamine clinic craze: Legalities and possibilities - canna law blog^{TM}. (n.d.). Harris Bricken. Retrieved March 22, 2021, from http://harrisbricken.com/cannalawblog/the-ketamine-clinic-craze-legalities-and-possibilities/

There are 3 types of ketamine—Which one works best? (2020, May 18). *DoubleBlind Mag*. https://doubleblindmag.com/there-are-3-types-of-ketamine-which-one-works-best/

Uptodate. (n.d.). Retrieved March 22, 2021, from https://www.uptodate.com/contents/ketamine-and-esketamine-for-treating-unipolar-depression-in-adults-administration-efficacy-and-adverse-effects

Wan, L.-B., Levitch, C. F., Perez, A. M., Brallier, J. W., Iosifescu, D. V., Chang, L. C., Foulkes, A., Mathew, S. J., Charney, D. S., & Murrough, J. W. (2015). Ketamine safety and tolerability in clinical trials for treatment-resistant depression. *The Journal of Clinical Psychiatry*, *76*(3), 247–252. https://doi.org/10.4088/JCP.13m08852

What is ptsd? (n.d.). Retrieved March 22, 2021, from https://www.psychiatry.org/patients-families/ptsd/what-is-ptsd

White, J. M., & Ryan, C. F. (1996). Pharmacological properties of ketamine. *Drug and Alcohol Review*, *15*(2), 145–155. https://doi.org/10.1080/09595239600185801

White, P. F., Ham, J., Way, W. L., & Trevor, A. J. (1980). Pharmacology of ketamine isomers in surgical patients. *Anesthesiology*, *52*(3), 231–239. https://doi.org/10.1097/00000542-198003000-00008

Wilkowska, A., Szałach, Ł., Słupski, J., Wielewicka, A., Czarnota, M., Gałuszko-Węgielnik, M., Wiglusz, M. S., & Cubała, W. J. (2020). Affective switch associated with oral, low dose ketamine treatment in a patient with treatment resistant bipolar i depression. Case report and literature review. *Frontiers in Psychiatry, 11.* https://doi.org/10.3389/fpsyt.2020.00516

Womble, A. L. (2013). Effects of ketamine on major depressive disorder in a patient with posttraumatic stress disorder. *AANA Journal, 81*(2), 118–119.

Wong, A., Benedict, N. J., Armahizer, M. J., & Kane-Gill, S. L. (2015). Evaluation of adjunctive ketamine to benzodiazepines for management of alcohol withdrawal syndrome. *Annals of Pharmacotherapy, 49*(1), 14–19. https://doi.org/10.1177/1060028014555859

Zanos, P., Moaddel, R., Morris, P. J., Georgiou, P., Fischell, J., Elmer, G. I., Alkondon, M., Yuan, P., Pribut, H. J., Singh, N. S., Dossou, K. S. S., Fang, Y., Huang, X.-P., Mayo, C. L., Wainer, I. W., Albuquerque, E. X., Thompson, S. M., Thomas, C. J., Zarate, C. A., & Gould, T. D. (2016). NMDAR inhibition-independent antidepressant actions of ketamine metabolites. *Nature, 533*(7604), 481–486. https://doi.org/10.1038/nature17998

Zhang, J.-C., Li, S.-X., & Hashimoto, K. (2014). R (-)-ketamine shows greater potency and longer lasting antidepressant effects than S (+)-ketamine. *Pharmacology, Biochemistry, and Behavior, 116,* 137–141. https://doi.org/10.1016/j.pbb.2013.11.033

Zhou, Y., & Danbolt, N. C. (2014). Glutamate as a neurotransmitter in the healthy brain. *Journal of Neural Transmission, 121*(8), 799–817. https://doi.org/10.1007/s00702-014-1180-8

Zimmerman, J. M., & Maren, S. (2010). NMDA receptor antagonism in the basolateral but not central amygdala blocks the extinction of Pavlovian fear conditioning in rats. *The European Journal of Neuroscience, 31*(9), 1664–1670. https://doi.org/10. 1/j.1460-9568.2010.07223.x

Zukauskaite, K. (n.d.). *The pros and cons of ketamine for obsessive compulsive disorder (Ocd)*. Stanford Medicine. Retrieved March 22, 2021, from http://stanmed.stanford.edu/2017summer/carolyn-rodriguez-ketamine-OCD.html

ACKNOWLEDGEMENTS

For the many wonderful people that picked me up and brushed me off.

Mom - Thank you for tirelessly defending, protecting, encouraging, and supporting me through all of life's ups and downs.

Marcie - Thank you for being my best friend, research buddy, and the person who inspires me to take action in health and in life.

Allen - Thank you for your generous help with my fundraiser and taking care of my sister.

Dad (Frank J.) and Uncle Clay (Clay L.) who both passed recently - Thank you guys for accepting and believing in me no matter what. I miss you both.

Aunt Bev - Thank you for sitting beside me in all of those doctors' office waiting rooms and telling me I'll be alright.

Aunt Diana - Thank you for driving me to so many doctor appointments and making sure I lack for nothing.

Aunt Judi - Thank you for always being a reliable source of support through thick and thin.

Suzanne - Thank you for sharing your personal and professional mental health experiences and always making me feel welcome.

Marissa - Thank you for being a great friend and teaching me to be a better one along the way.

Dr. and Mrs. Henry Macler - Thank you for opening the Ketamine clinic, saving my life, and offering an ongoing friendship of tremendous value.

Pittsburgh Ketamine clinic staff - Thank you Amy, Melissa, and Kerry for taking great care of me and making me feel like a part of the clinic's family.

The IOP staff at Allegheny Health Network, headed by Dr. Nancy Kennedy and complemented by Dr. Christina Smith, Jessica, and Vicky - Thank you for pulling me back from the edge.

Bruce Sorkin, PhD - Thank you for teaching me to deal with life head on and even laugh about it.

Amit Chopra, MD - Thank you for your sincere care and awesome expertise.

Vint Blackburn, MD - Thank you for counseling me through a shocking mystery illness we later learned was Hasimoto's Encephalitis.

Eric McDade, DO - Thank you for your patience with a frustrated, beleaguered patient, that led to the restoration of my brain and my life.

All nurses and staff of the "13th floor," at UPMC Western Psychiatric Institute - Thank you for watching over me tenderly when I was quite literally out of my mind.

So many family members and friends came through for me in my medical fundraiser several years ago. My bank account was at $0 due to my extraordinary medical bills. They funded my treatments when I saw 4 doctors/week.

Dean and Mary Marra - I can't thank you enough. I wish Uncle Bill was here to celebrate this. I miss him. He told me he'd be proud as long as I didn't turn out to be a lawyer!

Douglas and Tanita Ligons & Family
Dave and Rhonda Skiles & Family
Damon and Suzanne Skiles & Family
Nicole Rodgers-Provencher
PJ's Catering
Ray Zarzeczny
Allen Schwenk
Toni Czarnecki
Susan Foster Koval
Lisa DeBoe
Ed DeBoe
Ed Spix
Tony, Lynn & Marlene Denk

Keith & Jeanni Postlethwait

Ian Klock, DC - Thank you for applying your singular techniques to rebuilding my body from the devastation of an intense autoimmune disease.

Joseph Dimmateo, NMD, CCN, DHPh, RPh - Thank you friend, brother, and mentor for teaching me so much about health and for being a non-judgemental friend. I miss you.

Steven Handler, MD, PhD, CMD - Thank you for your personal and advisory support, without which I wouldn't have completed my Master's degree.

Rebecca Jacobson, MD, MS and Michael Becich, MD, PhD - Thank you for all of the wonderful opportunities in the Department of Biomedical Informatics within University of Pittsburgh's Medical School.

Wendy Chapman, PhD - Thank you for inviting me to graduate school and convincing me that I belonged there.

Daniel Resnick, PhD - Thank you for your mentorship in reading, writing, and research; skills that never go out of style.

Robert Mehrabian, PhD and Dr. Michael Murphy, PhD, MPM, M.Ed. - Thank you for a fantastic undergraduate education at Carnegie Mellon University.

Randy Blum - Thank you for seeing the potential in an unruly rebel.

Lisa Chin Mollica - Thank you for making my first online venture successful those many years ago. Without your talent and generosity, I never would have experienced the power of helping people online.

MKF for everything.

AUTHOR BIO

Frank M. Ligons holds a Master's of Science in Biomedical Informatics with co-authored research appearing in prestigious medical journals, including the Biomedical Journal of Quality & Safety, Journal of the American Medical Directors Association, and the American Medical Informatics Association® Proceedings.

He has presented medical research at the National Institutes of Health (NIH), National Library of Medicine (NLM), and the American Medical Informatics Association® Symposium (AMIA).

Mr. Ligons now specializes in exploring the benefits, safety, and payment strategies regarding Ketamine treatment in addressing mental, physical, and addiction-related illness. "The Ketamine Coach" writes regularly about low-dose Ketamine therapies at FindKetamine.com.

He lives in Pittsburgh, PA, eats raw eggs, and enjoys shared custody of his dog, Sticker.

Made in the USA
Middletown, DE
04 June 2022